Embracing Therapeutic Complexity

In an era where instant gratification has filtered into training programs geared toward technique-driven solutions, *Embracing Therapeutic Complexity* takes a step back and re-introduces fundamental touchstones that enable clinicians to apply an integrative treatment model in the service of in-depth healing and growth.

Using attachment theory as a bridge, this text connects key principles and practices that cut across various therapeutic disciplines and combines them into a unified framework where readers do not have to "put aside" their expertise in order to benefit from the skill sets provided in this book. In addition, this text addresses the impact that power and privilege have had on shaping our psychological constructs, and it challenges cultural assumptions and blind spots that have shaped our treatment approaches in the past.

Furthermore, this book illustrates how the application of psychodynamic principles can be combined with advances in trauma treatment, thus offering a practical guide for both beginning and seasoned therapists to amplify and expand their current clinical expertise.

Patricia Gianotti, Psy.D., is the Academic Director of The Institute for Advanced Psychotherapy at Loyola University Chicago and co-author of two earlier books, *Listening with Purpose* and *Uncovering the Resilient Core*.

"Finally, a panacea to the incompetence of manualized and technique-based approaches to treatment! This book is destined to become an invaluable training guide for developing solid psychotherapeutic integration skills that address the complexity and psychodynamic nuances of the contemporary patient. Dr. Gianotti's approach should be taught to every student of psychotherapy."

Jon Mills, *Psy.D., Ph.D., ABPP, Postgraduate Programs in Psychoanalysis & Psychotherapy, Adelphi University; Department of Psychosocial & Psychoanalytic Studies, University of Essex; Author of* Treating Attachment Pathology

"Psychoanalysis is not now, and has not been for decades, what many psychotherapists still think it is. Analysts today are centrally concerned with relationship, from the beginning of life, and attachment processes lie at the heart of the theory. Relational psychoanalysis has done much to promote these changes, and so this literature contributes directly and naturally to the general field of psychotherapy. Dr. Gianotti performs a great service by introducing relational psychoanalytic ideas to students and independent professionals who are interested in these ideas, but don't know how to find their way into them. She makes this introduction in the most practical way, presenting the material in a way that is sensitive to the changing realities of clinical practice, and to practitioners' uncertainty and worry about 'losing their way.' The book is full of clinical material and will be of interest both to those looking for a route of access into today's psychodynamic thinking and to psychoanalysts interested in contextualizing their work within the broader field of psychotherapy."

Donnel Stern, *Ph.D., Author,* The Infinity of the Unsaid: Unformulated Experience, Language, and the Nonverbal

"With this book, Patricia Gianotti offers a remedy for what ails current psychotherapies. Under pressure for quick fixes and inundated with modalities, today's therapists get lost and de-skilled. Gianotti suggests they ground themselves in certain complexities all therapies share, and she shows them how. She offers elegant big-picture maps that capture the interplay of self-expressive and shame-protective forces in patients' psychologies. She explains 'loyalty contracts' that block therapeutic progress. She argues for rigorous case conceptualization that includes patients' developmental and cultural contexts. A master clinician and teacher, Gianotti demonstrates how to drop down through language to right-brain moment-to-moment therapeutic presence, how to navigate psychic splits with delicate compassion, and how to finesse the power of transference for change. This is not a text on learning how to be a skillful relational psychodynamic practitioner, though it will serve that purpose well.

As Gianotti intends, it invites all practitioners into a big tent of understanding what they're doing, offering relief from confusion and self-doubt. With contextual understanding of their patients' suffering and permission to *slow the process down*, therapists can re-discover the healing connection that underpins all helpful interventions."

Patricia DeYoung, *MSW, Ph.D., Author*, Relational Psychotherapy: A Primer *and* Understanding and Treating Chronic Shame: Healing Right Brain Relational Trauma

"A 'must read' for student therapists and senior clinicians alike, Dr. Gianotti takes the rich cacophony of contemporary psychodynamic theory and creates her own unique synthesis. Clear, concise, and jargon-free, these concepts are now ready to be put to use in the clinical encounter. Her approach to psychodynamic formulation and understanding psychopathology are not pathologizing. Instead, Dr. Gianotti emphasizes how symptoms evolve and serve to protect and stabilize a fragile self. In addition she outlines specific clinical interventions, with abundant examples, that show how her psychodynamically-informed approach can help a therapist engage even those patients most resistant to change. This book is a great resource."

Rafael D. Ornstein, *M.D., Instructor in Psychiatry, Harvard Medical School*

"Dr. Gianotti has written a sophisticated, nuanced, scientifically based book that takes psychotherapy into the 21st century. This excellent volume provides practical guidance for new practitioners but has so much depth that even experienced therapists will return to it time and again when confronted with difficult situations that inevitably arise with complex patients. Kudos to Dr. Gianotti for integrating neuroscience, psychoanalysis, and evidence-based therapeutic techniques."

Barbara Ziv, *M.D., Adjunct Clinical Professor of Psychiatry, Temple University Medical School, Forensic Psychiatry expert for the prosecution in the Bill Cosby and Harvey Weinstein trials*

Embracing Therapeutic Complexity

A Guidebook to Integrating the Essentials of Psychodynamic Principles Across Therapeutic Disciplines

Patricia Gianotti

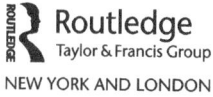

Routledge
Taylor & Francis Group

NEW YORK AND LONDON

Cover image: © Getty Images

First published 2022
by Routledge
605 Third Avenue, New York, NY 10158

and by Routledge
4 Park Square, Milton Park, Abingdon, Oxon, OX14 4RN

Routledge is an imprint of the Taylor & Francis Group, an informa business

© 2022 Patricia Gianotti

The right of Patricia Gianotti to be identified as author of this work has been asserted in accordance with sections 77 and 78 of the Copyright, Designs and Patents Act 1988.

Library of Congress Cataloguing-in-Publication Data
A catalog record for this title has been requested

ISBN: 978-0-367-63686-9 (hbk)
ISBN: 978-0-367-63685-2 (pbk)
ISBN: 978-1-003-12027-8 (ebk)

DOI: 10.4324/9781003120278

Typeset in Bembo
by MPS Limited, Dehradun

For Jack Danielian who gave birth to a vision
and
Jim Wayne who gave it wings to fly

Contents

List of Figures   xi
Foreword   xii
Acknowledgements   xv

Introduction: Designing a Framework That Connects
Attachment Theory, Neuropsychology, and Trauma
Treatment into a Psychodynamic Theoretical
Orientation   1

1   Creating a Three-Dimensional Matrix of the Psyche:
    Contrasting Two Roadmaps of Relational Development   21

2   Understanding the Power of Loyalty Contracts: How to
    Recognize, Articulate, and Interrupt Repeated Patterns
    of Early Relational Failures   49

3   Recasting the Art of Case Conceptualization: Holding
    the Macro and the Micro Perspective Within a Cultural
    Context   79

4   Getting Beneath the Tip of the Iceberg: How to Use
    Entry Points in Language to Uncover Hidden Material   109

5   Mastering the Technique of Moment-to-Moment
    Tracking: Mirroring, Sequential Reflection, and
    Reframing   129

6 Speaking to the Splits: Understanding the Continuum of
Dissociative Process   154

7 Working with Transferential Enactments as a Leverage
for Change   188

Index   224

Figures

1.1	Two Model Comparison	25
1.2	The Four Quadrant Model	29
1.3	Healthy Self-Actualization Model	34
1.4	The Four Quadrant Model	36
1.5	Healthy Self-Actualization Model	36
2.1	Quid Pro Quo Formula	55
3.1	Underlying Factors that Create Vulnerability	86
3.2	The Four Quadrant Model	93
4.1	Getting Beneath the Tip of the Iceberg	118
4.2	Start with the Entry Point: Track the Dialogue	121
4.3	Client's Internal Dialogue	123
4.4	Continued Tracking of Entry Points	124
4.5	Analyzing the Learning with Clients	126
4.6	Practice Toward Mastery	127
5.1	Vicious Pain Cycle	136
5.2	Kathy's Triggers	140
5.3	Ben's Triggers	141
6.1	The Four Quadrant Model	162

Foreword

In an era in which the evolution of our profession looks increasingly – and depressingly – like capitalism on steroids; in which ambitious therapeutic entrepreneurs generate an ever proliferating volume of what are essentially "startups," each with its own acronymed brand and claims of unique virtues that differentiate it from the almost identical brands offered by the competition; in which intellectual silos impede learning from those working on related problems across artificial theoretical, institutional, or organizational divides, Patricia Gianotti has the temerity to offer a book that aims to present psychodynamic principles in ways that make sense to therapists of all orientations, to show how the different perspectives in our field *intersect* rather than clash, how therapists of different backgrounds can learn from each other and build on each other's innovations and insights rather than treating product differentiation as the highest value. As the very title of the book signals, she is interested in *complexity*, rather than in promoting an acronymed brand.

In pursuing this aim, Gianotti brings an openness to diverse ideas and a commitment to helping people change broadly and deeply, not just symptomatically, that is increasingly rare in a quick-fix society. Her vision is broad and integrative, pulling together ideas and methods from a wide variety of sources, but she is particularly focused on exploring the implications of neurobiological research, attachment phenomena, and the impact of trauma. Weaving these themes together in a framework that highlights the ways human beings develop and live in *relationships*, and how the therapeutic effort too must be grounded in an appreciation of its fundamentally relational foundations, Gianotti offers a vision of the therapeutic process that provides new insights and refinements for the psychodynamic therapist as well as valuable enhancements and points of entry for the therapist trained in other points of view.

As in her previous two books, written with the late Jack Danielian (Danielian & Gianotti, 2012, Gianotti & Danielian, 2017), Gianotti is keenly sensitive to the experience and dynamics of shame. Shame, as a central and powerful force both in the course of our development and in generating and maintaining the problems that bring people to therapy, was a rather late addition to the conceptual foundations of therapeutic practice and theory and is still insufficiently integrated into the thinking of therapists of many orientations. Gianotti and Danielian were important contributors to the deepening of our understanding of its impact and dynamics, and in this new book, Patricia Gianotti advances this understanding still further. She offers innovative ways of working with the dynamics of shame and further understanding of its intimate and intricate connections with attachment phenomena, social as well as interpersonal dynamics, and the very nature of the way the brain is wired.

I was first drawn to Gianotti's (and Danielian's) work through my interest in Karen Horney. Horney has seemed to me one of the most important of the "forgotten" theorists in our field, a thinker whose insights preceded and pointed to much in the contemporary relational movement, but who is rarely acknowledged as one of its foundational forerunners. Like Gianotti, Horney eschewed obscurantistic technical language. She wrote in a crystal clear, transparent English that, in itself, probably contributed to her not being widely or enduringly regarded as of the very first rank of psychoanalytic thinkers and writers, a category to which I strongly believe she belongs. The very clarity and simplicity of her prose made it hard for many to regard what she was saying as being as profound and genuinely innovative as I believe it was. Paradoxically, she was dismissed as a lightweight while shunned as a dangerous challenger to received psychoanalytic ideas. It has always also struck me as a fascinating irony that Horney, who grew up in Germany, wrote crystal clear English at a time when many American-born analysts wrote a version of English that at times read more like it was German. This present book by Gianotti does not as directly display its connection to Horney's work as her earlier books, but as I read it, it develops in new ways many of the original Horney-inspired themes that characterized Gianotti's earlier work. And it continues to share Horney's commitment to avoid jargon and technical language wherever possible.

One particularly important way in which Gianotti continues and further develops her earlier ties to Horney's work is in her attention to culture and society. Horney was one of the earliest psychoanalytic writers to genuinely take culture and society seriously, not as a simple projection of inner drives and fantasies (e.g., Horney, 1937), and to the degree that she continues to be studied today, it is this emphasis that is one of the most central points of interest. Gianotti's longstanding rooting in Horney's thought, among other influences, is evident in her focus on the critical role of culture and society in shaping both the strengths and the weaknesses evident in the patterns discernible in our patients' lives. Especially noteworthy is the attention she gives to experiences both of privilege and marginalization.

Horney's influence is also evident in Gianotti's strong emphasis on staying with what is happening in the present, on not utilizing the real and important insights about the impact of early experiences that she offers as an excuse to retreat from the present. Horney's *New Ways in Psychoanalysis* (Horney, 1939) was a brilliant and powerful critique of the way that psychoanalysis to that point had regarded the present as a mere repetition or representation, failing to appreciate the *evolving* nature of personality and the ways in which what is happening in the present really *matters*, is not a mere screen for the past. Gianotti pursues this same path, pointing out that "For those who are psychoanalytically trained, if what is unfolding in the present moment is only understood as a reflection of past fixations, the present is eclipsed by the past and nuances of change or growth can be missed." Tying this emphasis not only to Horney but to Stern's (2004) highlighting of the importance of the present moment in psychotherapy and to a further range of developmental theorists who view development *as* development, as continuing in a dynamic, reciprocal intersubjective manner throughout life rather than as fixated or arrested in a purely internal fashion, Gianotti aims for a therapeutic approach that is keenly attentive both to the impact of the past and the emotional reality of the present. She has offered us an important contribution to the theoretical and clinical literature

Paul L. Wachtel, Ph.D.,
Distinguished Professor,
Doctoral Program in Clinical Psychology,
City College of New York

References

Danielian, J., & Gianotti, P. (2012). *Listening with purpose: Entry points into shame and narcissistic vulnerability*. Plymouth, UK: Jason Aronson.

Gianottti, P., & Danielian, J. (2017). *Uncovering the resilient core: A workbook on the treatment of narcissistic defeneses, shame, and emerging authenticity*. New York: Routledge.

Horney, K. (1937). *The neurotic personality of our time*. New York: Norton.

Horney, K. (1939). *New ways in psychoanalysis*. New York: Norton.

Stern, D. N. (2004). *The present moment in psychotherapy and everyday life*. New York: Norton.

Acknowledgements

The inspiration for writing this book came from years of working with a team of dedicated colleagues who have been part of an advanced, year-long certificate program designed to expand the proficiency of licensed professionals from various clinical disciplines. Our collaborative process helped us design a curriculum that was structured but also left room for fluidity in our thinking as we continually adapted our knowledge base to keep up with the evolving changes in our field. This book represents a consolidation of our observations and teaching methods as they were shaped and modified by student feedback over the years. Translating theory into applied practice is no simple task. Translating theory into practices that can be utilized by practitioners who come from a wide variety of clinical orientations is what makes theory become universally useful and alive.

In the beginning stages of writing, colleagues who read my early chapters repeatedly asked, "Now, who is your audience?" I wanted to say *everyone*, even though I realized this might be an overly ambitious reach. Their question, however, did force me to become clearer about my intentions. What I *did* know was that I wanted to publish an integrative, psychodynamically oriented text that used language in such a way that complex subject matter could be understood by *any* clinician, regardless of their theoretical orientation or years of experience. I also knew that I wanted to integrate advances in neurobiological research as they pertained to attachment injuries and the treatment of trauma and incorporate those advances into a working model that was fluid enough to hold the richness of both psychodynamic and neurobiological areas of scholarship.

This meant that the material in this text had to be sophisticated enough to be of interest to seasoned professionals, but not so academically dense that it would run the risk of losing therapists who were not familiar with psychodynamic terminology. Based on my experience as the director of a training institute, I have had the opportunity to encounter a wide spectrum of graduates and licensed professionals, the majority of whom had received no formal training in relationally-based psychodynamic theory. Through this experience I also began to realize that the richness and value of psychodynamic principles were on the verge of becoming so diminished that they were no longer used by larger and larger numbers of practitioners. Even though dynamic practice had made enormous advances in the past twenty years, I wondered if we were about to become a dying breed. This created a sense of urgency in me. I wanted to convey the value of psychodynamic theory in a way that non-dynamically trained therapists could not only understand and appreciate these foundational principles but also integrate them into their own areas of expertise.

My hope is that readers will find this text understandable and *hands-on enough* so that the macro-picture of psychodynamic principles can be applied to the micro-clinical moment of day-to-day practice. My goal was to capture the experience of what it is like to sit in the room with a patient hour after hour and to then provide guidance around common stumbling blocks when therapists feel stuck or struggle to find words as to what to say next. I also wanted to create a unifying roadmap that therapists could use, regardless of their clinical experience and orientation. My further goal was to present a picture of the figure and the ground of case analysis in a way that could be applied cross-culturally as well. And yet, I didn't want the book to turn into something so simplistic or formulaic that readers would be left feeling as if they were being asked to follow a cookie-cutter recipe for clinical practice.

The scope of the book is comprehensive, highlighting new perspectives on trauma treatment and attachment theory. For newer clinicians this book offers a compelling framework in which to organize and craft comprehensive treatment plans, and it is particularly useful in identifying and understanding transferential enactments and counter-transferential reactions. For seasoned therapists, this book offers an integration of neurobiological findings into psychodynamic frameworks, as well as considering the effects that social privilege and marginalization have had on shaping personality development. Expanding what we frame as important as well as challenging routinized assumptions are evolving parts of the learning curve throughout one's clinical career.

It takes a legion of support to complete a book. Multiple eyes on the project are what shaped it into a finished product. I want to give special thanks to two of my dear friends and colleagues, Donna Knudsen and LR Berger who painstakingly read, edited, and made important additions to each and every chapter. They also lent me their expertise in the area of understanding the neurobiological impact of attachment injury as it pertains to the treatment of trauma. I also extend my deep appreciation and thanks to my valued colleague, Alana Tappin, who helped me expand my thinking around issues of diversity, power, privilege and cultural marginalization. Her wisdom and perspective included important additions throughout this text, but her contributions to Chapter Three were particularly valuable in terms of understanding the importance of cultural marginalization when it comes to crafting a psychodynamic case formulation. Thanks also goes to my colleague, Richard Raubolt, who engaged me in rigorous thought and gave me critical feedback as well as ongoing encouragement along the way

My deepest appreciation goes to my husband, Stephen Gianotti, whose patience, steady counsel, and generous spirit allowed me the time and support I needed to complete this book. My heart-felt gratitude and thanks go to Paul Wachtel for writing the Foreword to this book. He has been a mentor and an example of professionalism and generosity to many of us in the field. The clarity of his theoretical contributions and his wisdom have become an integral part of my own writing style and how I engage in the therapeutic relational process. Grateful thanks go to Donnel Stern, Patricia DeYoung, Jon Mills, Rafael Ornstein, and Barbara Ziv who graciously wrote endorsements for this book. Finally, I wish to thank my editors at Routledge, Sarah Gore, Upasruti Biswas, and Abigail Stanley whose guidance and timely responses were most appreciated.

Donna Knudsen, Alana Tappin, Bob Taseff, Jacqui Casey, Jim Wayne, Maria Scharfenberger, and the entire faculty at The Institute of Advanced Psychotherapy at Loyola University Chicago as well as each and every student who participated in our year-long program over the years helped give birth to this book. Our interaction around clinical material specifically helped us revise our thinking as to how to best convey complex teaching methods to help bring theoretical concepts to life. Credit for the graphic designs contained within this text go to Tiffany Bishop, whose patience and attention to detail was invaluable. Finally, I could not have done any of this without my valued colleague and administrative assistant, Katelyn Tippett, a woman who is worth her weight in gold. As copy editor, proofreader, and advisor, she was there with me every step of the way.

Introduction: Designing a Framework That Connects Attachment Theory, Neuropsychology, and Trauma Treatment into a Psychodynamic Theoretical Orientation

Rationale for This Book

This book is aimed at helping therapists from various clinical disciplines to further integrate psychodynamic principles and techniques into their treatment approach. My hope is that non-dynamically trained therapists will see the value in incorporating key principles of psychodynamic therapy into their practice as a way to broaden their skill sets. My further hope is that therapists who *are* dynamically trained will see this text as a roadmap offering both *a set of unifying principles* within the broad scope of dynamic theory and *an integrative method* of incorporating contributions from other areas of clinical exploration, namely, neurobiological research findings that have advanced strategic interventions around complex trauma and early attachment injury. These domains of clinical research and practice are reshaping how we treat individuals who show varying degrees of affect dysregulation and more severe symptomatic and behavioral psychopathology.

Relationally based dynamic approaches have been scientifically validated by current discoveries in neurobiology. Specifically, these studies relate to how one's sense of self develops within the constructs of human interpersonal relationship, and most importantly, the centrality of relationship in repairing early relational attachment injuries. Through the application of these hard-wired components of neurological development, we can see how the natural capacity of the mind to heal in relationship is activated by attending to the relational principles of psychodynamic theory.

This book is also aimed at drawing attention to a fairly dramatic shift in focus that has occurred in graduate mental health programs across the country. Over the past two decades, pressure from managed-care insurance companies to reduce the allotted time for reimbursable mental health treatment has resulted in graduate schools shifting their curricula to short-term treatment models in an effort to "prepare" their graduates for the realities of 21st-century practice. Unfortunately, course offerings including psychodynamic models that offered a more complete understanding of what it means to enter into the dynamic complexities of a therapeutic

DOI: 10.4324/9781003120278-1

relationship were often eliminated. I, and other colleagues who coordinate advanced training programs for licensed post-graduate professionals across the country, have found that the impact of these changes has left students underprepared in terms of grasping the depth and breadth of knowledge that is necessary for those entering today's workplace, particularly within treatment settings that are geared to the underserved populations and those patients who present with more severe psychopathology.

My colleagues and I universally have found that this generation of practitioners seems to have varying degrees of difficulty grasping the "big picture" of therapeutic complexity. That is, we have observed that newly trained clinicians often attempt a variety of techniques without necessarily knowing what impact these techniques will have on a patient or why they are choosing a particular intervention at any given point in time. We believe that this may be one of the unfortunate outcomes of graduate training that is too narrowly focused on mastering techniques rather than on having a solid grounding in case conceptualization. This, coupled with managed-care insurance mandates, seems to have resulted in a pressure to "fix" patient problems in 8–12 sessions or less. Many of today's treatment interventions seem to be exclusively geared to psychoeducation, cognitive-behavioral strategies, or solution-focused treatments aimed at symptom reduction. Often, when these methods don't produce immediate results, or when patients quickly relapse, therapists, especially beginning therapists, eventually began to feel somewhat lost or demoralized (see Hazanov, 2019).

The feeling of *losing one's way*, that point of clinical uncertainty, can manifest in a variety of ways – as confusion around what to say next, as an internal pressure to prove one's competence, as an attempt to hold onto one's theoretical framework too tightly, or as self-doubt about whether therapeutic progress is being made. It is in these moments of uncertainty that therapists are most vulnerable to losing their clinical flexibility, either by trying to lead the client, by making assumptions or untimely interpretations, or by over-using a technique in a way that says, "one size fits all". In turn these clinical missteps often leave clients feeling confused, cut off, judged, even humiliated. Teaching clinicians how to follow rather than lead, how to trust in the unfolding process, how to slow down the pace enough so that clients feel seen, safe, and supported is the terrain where some of the most difficult and delicate work of complex short or long-term therapy occurs. The aim of this book is to provide a process-oriented approach of how to enter and navigate the scope of delicate and deep listening.

Creating a Method that can be Replicated Across Disciplines

Long-term psychodynamic constructs are teachable and replicable, but only if a methodology is provided for how to think about what we see and what we hear in the unfolding present. Understanding how to integrate theoretical constructs with the evolving clinical observations is precisely how clinicians can become more comfortable with the unfolding process dynamics within the treatment hour. Rather than using extended theoretical elaboration, this book breaks from complicated psychodynamic language and jargon often found in academic texts. Instead, it presents a visual graphic model that identifies component parts of the psyche and then analyzes how these parts connect to other parts of the evolving self. When patients initially enter into therapy, some parts of the self are presented in the patient's conscious narrative; other parts, however, are hidden from view, and still other parts remain unknown or unformulated. Through analyzing how these various aspects of the psyche are integrated or split off from the whole is critically important if we are to become more adept at creating entry points into deeper communication, as well as creating leverage points that allow us to dismantle defense structures, repair traumatic injuries, and free-up our clients' innate capacities.

Toward that end, this text provides the clinicians with a three-fold approach to examining and understanding complex "sticking points" in treatment that focuses on a combination of: (a) dynamic formulation, (b) practice techniques, and (c) a model that can be applied across multiple theoretical orientations. Through in-depth clinical illustrations, the reader is provided with a road map, a set of organizing principles that offer a unifying bridge across many theoretical schools of thought. Additionally, this text offers a methodology for breaking through repeated enactments that reflect traumatic or dysfunctional beliefs and relational patterns. Various chapters will illustrate specific examples of listening, tracking, and intervention techniques that can be incorporated into a clinician's existing theoretical orientation or area of clinical expertise. In addition, because this book focuses primarily on clinical application, terms often associated with psychodynamic theory have been translated into practice intervention strategies that can be understood across disciplines.

Although the theoretical grounding of this text is based on a psychodynamic approach, this book draws heavily upon principles based in attachment theory as a way of illustrating how learned attachment styles create repeating patterns in adulthood, patterns that often reflect deep-seated longings, fears, and assumptions. Two models of the psyche are provided, one that reflects healthy self-development, and one that is defensively constructed to hide underlying feelings of shame and inadequacy. Both models, in turn, offer a three-dimensional picture that draws attention to intrapsychic, relational, and socio-cultural aspects of human strengths, resources, and vulnerabilities. These concise graphics allow for a comparison of healthy and defensive attempts at adaptation. Used as an assessment tool throughout the therapeutic process, these models enable therapists to more easily identify how the various personal components of a person interact to form a fluid vs. more rigid homeostatic balance. The complexity of each individual's unique personal make-up includes the parts of the self that are healthy and adaptive, and parts of the self that operate from defensively driven reactivity. The degree of health and defensive reactivity can be more clearly seen and assessed by contrasting these two models of learned attachment styles and consequent approaches toward adaptation.

What contemporary psychodynamic training offers practitioners is a way of *thinking about* the complexity of the psyche from a variety of lenses and as way of simultaneously attending to multiple dimensions of what we are observing. As the Academic Director of The Institute for Advanced Psychotherapy at Loyola University Chicago, an advanced certificate program for licensed therapists, my colleagues and I have observed that clinicians from a wide range of therapeutic disciplines have found great benefit from incorporating the basic underpinnings of psychodynamic theory into their practice. What our trainees universally have brought to the learning process is a hunger for being able to use a method of understanding cases from a "big picture" context. Many of our clinician-trainees seem to be missing an over-arching framework that anchors and guides their strategies. Because of this gap, trainees often had difficulty assessing the level of rigidity or stability of the patient's psychic structure and often felt stuck as to where to go or what to say next.

The Value of Applying Psychodynamic Principles – What Got Lost

In our view, comprehensive treatment also involves an understanding of the past couple of decades, in large measure because non-dynamically trained practitioners do not necessarily understand how psychodynamic theory has changed over the past two decades. Classical analysis, which was primarily based on drive theory, has shifted to a more relational approach, one that is a two-person psychology, where both parties – the therapist and the client – bring their subjective experience into the relational mix. In addition, psychodynamic therapy has been greatly enriched by the contributions of trauma treatment, attachment theory, and neuropsychological advances that have helped us shift our attentional focus from conflicts based on past fixations, to a focus on trusting that any unresolved issues from the past will manifest in the present moment within the container of the treatment relationship.

Contemporary psychodynamic models help see the big picture by identifying the various puzzle pieces that comprise the complex workings of the human psyche. Dynamic therapy attends to how patients organize their thoughts as well as how accurately patients are able to read and monitor levels of comfort or discomfort within feeling states. As is the case with most therapeutic models, psychodynamic treatment is centered first and foremost on creating a safe relational container in order that the therapeutic process can optimally unfold.

Unlike other theoretical orientations that focus on techniques aimed at ameliorating acute symptom relief, psychodynamic models believe that the dynamic interaction between the patient and the therapist is of utmost importance, which is why working with transference and counter-transference is a critical leverage point in the change process. Whether you have been trained in working with transference or not, all therapeutic re-lationships evoke some degree of transferential dynamics. Understanding and anticipating transferential triggers can improve any treatment outcome, regardless of your orientation or training background, regardless of whether you do short- or long-term therapy, regardless of your area of clinical specialization.

The art of case conceptualization, a critically useful skill set for both short and long-term treatment modalities, is one of the major foundation stones of psychodynamic practice that seems to have gotten lost in many training institutions. Case formulation provides clinicians with a way to think about *the complexity of interconnected parts of the personality*, rather than training them to think about an *intervention strategy or technique*. Therapists who haven't been taught how to conceptualize a dynamic formulation are at a dis-advantage because they often have a difficult time analyzing how the var-ious and parts of the patient's psyche fit or do not fit into a congruent narrative. To hold the complexity of what is required to enter into the deeper waters of long-term treatment means that we must attend not only to providing our patients with symptom relief, but we also need to un-derstand the etiology of their symptoms from multiple vantage-points – from examining the quality of their attachment, to the rigidity or flexibility of their behaviors, beliefs, and relational patterns, to their expectations of self and other, to assessing their capacity for self-reflection, and their ca-pacity to assimilate new information.

Comprehensive treatment also involves an understanding of process dynamics. To assess and track the quality and strength of the therapeutic relationship as it evolves over time, the therapist must have the ability to move in and closely attend to the nuance of what a client is trying to communicate while simultaneously keeping in awareness the patient's over-arching vulnerabilities, repeated patterns, as well as what interventions may trigger defensive reactivity. The ability to hold both macro- and micro-clinical observations simultaneously is precisely how clinicians deepen the therapeutic relationship and become more comfortable with unfolding the process dynamics within the treatment hour. Often therapists err in one direction or the other. They either over-attend to content and problem solving and therefore try to rush the process because they have difficulty assessing the core stability or fragility of their patients. Or they over-attend to history, diagnosis, and theoretical constructs, which runs the risk of having the therapist's own assumptions color what he/she hears, thus running the risk of missing subtle communication cues that could open new doorways of seeing and understanding the patient's uniqueness.

Underlying Principles

An emerging interest in the field of psychotherapeutic research and practice is centered on identifying and measuring key principles and techniques that are effective within and across the major theoretical disciplines. The APA is in a collaborative endeavor with professionals and trainees around the world to test and research the acquisition of therapy skill set and have just begun the first in a series of testing the essentials of deliberate practice within each of the major disciplines. Other practitioners from The Society for the Exploration of Psychotherapy Integration (SEPI) and the National Institute for the Psychotherapies (NIP) are dedicated to exploring ways to find commonalities across disciplines and to introduce outside interventions into relational analytic therapy. The interest these organization have in identifying essential skill sets within each major discipline can also act as an invitation to open up dialogue across therapeutic disciplines in search of commonalities, a cross-pollination of practice techniques in the service of producing more favorable therapeutic outcomes. This text presents both a method and compilation of techniques drawn from a number of theoretical orientations in the spirit of therapeutic integration.

Toward that end, neuropsychologically based interventions are increasingly seen as offering valuable, observation-based data based on infant research, specifically observations of early infant–parent interactions. These observations and conclusions around relational conditions that produce a secure attachment can be applied to psychological treatment with both child and adult populations, thanks to multiple contributors in the field whose findings span over 50 decades (Beebe et al., 2010; Beebe & Lachmann, 1988; Frank & LaBarre, 2010; Lyons-Ruth, 1998, 1999; Lyons-Ruth et al., 2006; Pally, 1998, 2000; Stern et al., 1998, Tronick, 1998). Their studies verify the conclusions of early attachment theorists (Ainsworth, 1964, 1967; Ainsworth & Bell, 1970; Ainsworth & Bowlby, 1991; Bowlby, 1951). Infant–parent researchers all speak to the importance of identifying conditions and factors that create a secure attachment. Current research observations between a parent and children, prior to the development of language, can predict individuals who will experience dissociative episodes in later life (Cyr et al., 2010; Dutra et al., 2009; Ogawa et al., 1997). Learning to listen to the affective resonance of our clients and noticing where dissociative ruptures occur within treatment is critical to the healing process around early attachment injuries. Phillip Bromberg was known to say that the body's mind speaks its own affective language; the more one can listen to it affectively, the more fluent the body's language becomes in communicating what it knows.

Marvin Goldfried, in his search to obtain consensus in practices across the three major disciplines in psychotherapy, observed that the three major orientations are psychodynamic, cognitive-behavioral, and experiential/humanistic orientation. He states, "Common principles, rather than abstract theoretical orientations or specific techniques is where the field may discover consensus across schools of therapy" (2019, p. 487). Goldfried, whose clinical orientation is primarily cognitive/behavioral, identifies the following principles of change (1982, 2019, p. 488):

- Promoting client expectation and motivation that therapy can help,
- Establishing an optimal therapeutic alliance,
- Facilitating client awareness of the factors associated with his or her difficulties,
- Encouraging the client to engage in corrective experiences, and
- Emphasizing ongoing reality testing in the client's life.

Stephen Mitchell reminds us that we must continually challenge ourselves around our theoretical approach by asking ourselves – *What does the patient need?* and *What does the therapist know?* Rather than our theoretical training governing what dictates our interventional strategies, remaining curious as to what the patient needs in order to repair old wounds is a stance that ensures a continual stretching of our clinical thinking and intersubjective curiosity.

Leo Stone (1961), an early classical analyst, had written a courageous book, *The Psychoanalytic Situation*. Stone, who preceded Mitchell's writing, challenged the classical analytic orthodoxy of his era by arguing that technique *must be* tailored to the patient. Even early analysts, Ferenczi (1919), Ferenczi and Rank (1925), and Alexander and French (1946), challenged Freud's analytic technique and the centrality of the Oedipal complex, and began advocating exploring and adapting psychoanalytic techniques to fit the needs of the patient.

Paul Wachtel reminds us that our theoretical assumptions and predilections influence what observations we make and which ones we don't even think to make. Our assumptions influence *what we see,* even when we choose to look in a certain direction, and they also affect *how we interpret* or make sense of what we see. In other words, our theories influence what the data are as well as how we intervene around the data based on those assumptions.

Unifying Principles within Relational Psychodynamic Practice

Unifying principles within relational psychodynamic practice begins with the foundation of creating a solid and safe therapeutic relationship. By creating a safe container, therapist and client are able to explore and resolve past relational injuries, uncover repressed memories that inhibit growth and development, discover aspects of the self that were either disavowed or unknown. This, in turn, creates an environment and process where the client's resilience and authenticity begin to emerge, where together they can explore and set inspirational, yet realistic goals in terms of maximizing the client's unique potential as well as creating mutually satisfying relationships with others in the outside world.

Theoretical areas that help to facilitate these processes are:

- A grounding in attachment theory and an ability to assess the individual's quality of early attachments as they impact present functioning, including *yearning for reparation* as well as ingrained *fear and mistrust* that relationships will result in hurt, betrayal, and disappointment.
- An understanding that neuroscience has documented that the quality of the relationship between caretaker and child significantly impacts the development of the limbic system and thereby the capacity and ability to regulate affect that can be mitigated and restructured through optimal relational therapeutic interventions.
- An understanding that attachment needs are hard-wired and include the expectation that verbal and nonverbal communication cues will elicit a matching response. This pattern, which we call the *serve and return*, inform the therapist–client response patterns.
- An understanding of the concept of *figure and ground* (holding the micro and the macro attention) when it comes to case conceptualization, including the development of an initial as well as an evolving working hypothesis of what is unfolding in the treatment at any given point in time.
- An understanding that the internalization of shame is an outcome and the residue of early attachment damage, as well as later traumatic experiences, and it plays out in relational dynamics both consciously and unconsciously.
- An acknowledgement that internalized shame is also produced and reinforced by cultural norms and values based on inclusion and marginalization and that our evolving understanding of treatment must embrace an openness and curiosity around culture, context, as well as an acknowledgement of theoretical assumptions and blind spots.
- A working knowledge of transference and countertransference dynamics along with an expertise and comfort with witnessing and processing unfolding dynamics during the course of therapy, grounded in the knowledge that all unfinished historical material plays out in the present moment.
- An acknowledgement that one aspect of the therapeutic healing process occurs through the relational dynamic of *disruption and repair*, that is, disruption in the therapeutic relationship also creates a powerful

opportunity to repair the disruption, thus changing old patterns around disappointment and mistrust.

- An understanding that resilience is an innate aspect of the human spirit, and even in individuals with histories of severe trauma or deprivation, the seeds of resilience lie at the core of the self.

How This Text Addresses Each of the Above Theoretical Principles and Practices

I   In two previous books written with my co-author, Jack Danielian, *Listening with Purpose* (2012) and *Uncovering the Resilient Core* (2017), we designed a model and a treatment approach that addresses key principles and practices within the wide umbrella of psychodynamic treatment. We introduced a graphic, called the Four Quadrant Model, which is a visual matrix that provides a snapshot of multiple psychological dimensions and dynamics of the personality simultaneously, ones that attend to intrapsychic, relational, systemic, and culture theoretical constructs. Essentially, this graphic illustrates a means by which therapists can visualize how parts of the psyche are either integrated, minimized, or defensively split off from a patient's conscious narrative.

The model is designed to capture a picture of strategies and organizing schemas that people develop as a result of having suffered varying degrees of relational injury in childhood. The four quadrants show the relationship between learned defense patterns resulting from early attachment failures and how they shape the development of beliefs, fears, and longings around self-achievement, relational expectations of others, and repeating response patterns once an individual experiences disappointment in self or others. Because children will do anything to preserve the precarious attachment with parental figures, authentic self-development is often sacrificed to regain a sense of safety. Therefore, the Four Quadrant Model represents a picture of learned strategies the psyche reflexively develops in the service of psychological protection from danger or psychic fragmentation.

Learned defense mechanisms have somewhat predictable patterns, which function in the service of achieving and maintaining psychic stability and coherence. Karen Horney (1950) states that people's relational style falls into three basic modes of engaging with others in the world. Individuals either adopt a basic positional stance of:

- moving *toward* others, by seeking connection and accommodation,
- moving *away* from others, by adopting a position of freedom, independence, and avoidance of any limitation imposed by society,
- or moving *against* others, by establishing dominance and superiority over others.

Neurobiological evidence has shown that there are limited possibilities of patterns of human behavior based on the composition of our nervous systems. For example, we are hard-wired for connection, neurobiological systems shut down in the face of severe trauma or neglect, and neurobiological development is relational, in that early attachment templates are encoded right-brain-to-right-brain that impact overall brain development (Schore, 2012, 2016, 2019). Horney's description of the aforementioned character solutions illustrates three basic patterns of behavior based on early encoded relational patterns that attempt to regulate and maintain feelings of self-worth and self-stabilization when attachment fractures occur within the parent–child bond. Although Horney's descriptors are elegant in their simplicity, they are not meant to be seen as reductionist in terms of our understanding of the complex variations of human dynamics. The more parts of the complex picture of the psyche we can grasp an incorporate into our theoretical models, the better we will become at developing intervention strategies.

This text will elaborate on concepts presented through the Four Quadrant Model illustrating how to use this model in part-whole analysis around case conceptualization throughout the treatment process. In addition, a new model will be introduced, called the Healthy Self-Actualizing Model, which provides a picture of the evolving psychic development of the self and the self in relationship throughout the life span. This model presents a picture of what secure attachment looks like in childhood and how healthy connection allows for authentic, unrestricted emergence and growth. These two models can be used as an assessment tool, assisting the therapist throughout the treatment process. In addition, the Four Quadrant Model connects defense mechanisms of over-compensation, splitting, and retaliation as attempts to keep feelings of shame at bay. In this sense, the model can be viewed as an attempt to create homeostatic balance and self-regulation.

II   A second way this text addresses unifying theoretical principles and practices is by stressing the importance of *slowing down* the dialogic process. Slowing down the process is both a therapeutic stance as well as a technique. When therapists introduce a change of pace in response to a client's reporting of feelings or events, this can have a fairly immediate impact on the client's ability to slow themselves down, whether that be consciously or unconsciously. You will notice that breathing patterns begin to change. Clients often will become more "present" and connected, making eye contact, or they may become self-reflective, all of which can calm anxiety and increase the capacity for self-regulation of affect.

Intentionally slowing our own responses down can interrupt automatic, habituated thoughts and reactions on the part of the patient as well as ourselves. This can open the doorway for therapist and client to join in identifying automatic assumptions that may have led to high degrees of agitation. Or it can create an invitation to become more curious about alternative ways of responding, where the therapist and client can engage in a dialogue that allows for the examination of fixed beliefs and expectations, connecting these beliefs and assumptions to repeated patterns of disappointment, over-achievement, or feelings of hopelessness in adulthood.

By asking questions that encourage patients to fill in the details of their life story in greater depth, we are demonstrating a quality of attention that is both respectful and gentle. It is a way of being with the client that non-verbally conveys a message that we believe that what the client has to say is important. It is a way that our patients begin to relax and develop more trust in us and in the therapeutic process. Out of this container of therapeutic safety, patients will eventually begin to recount painful memories or discover pockets of resilience that are finally being given permission to emerge. It is also a way for transferential reenactments to emerge and be explored. If the therapist slows her own pace down during these moments, it lessens the chance of making quick judgment, preemptive interpretations, or counter-transferential reactivity on the part of the therapist.

When therapists bring careful attention to the moment-to-moment interaction in the unfolding present, they are engaging with the patient in an intersubjective, non-hierarchical process, where what is emerging can be explored as a shared enterprise. In between the lines, by slowing the process down, the therapist is conveying that the patient has what it takes to uncover hidden material, dismantle feelings of shame and inadequacy, challenge parental assumptions and beliefs, and discover the wisdom that lies within the core of the self. With multiple repetitions, this quality of attention, the internalization of the rhythm of the dynamic exchange becomes internalized. A new relational process can then become encoded in memory, to be used again and again as a self-reflective capacity.

III A third way this text addresses unifying theoretical principles and practices is by conceptualizing the process of psychotherapy in the present moment. Daniel Stern (2004) states that the longer the therapist can stay with the present moment and explore what unfolds, the more different paths to pursue will open up. If viewed micro-analytically with the present moment and sequences of present moments as the focus, one starts to see it unfolding somewhat differently than we usually do. By staying in the present moment, our understanding of process moves closer to the foreground, and the search for meaning moves more to the background. The result is a greater appreciation of experience, and a less-hurried rush to interpretation (p. 28).

I would describe this shift as moving from being theory bound to observation bound. Errors in how interventions are made can be made either by trying to lead the client into the past or pushing the client into the future. For those who have primarily been trained in addressing symptom relief, the temptation is to lead a client forward to help "fix" the problem. This can occur by over-using techniques that avoid emersion into painful feeling states or speaking to logic and intellect through the use of psychoeducation. If what is unfolding in the present moment contains painful affect or uncomfortable content, the therapist may be tempted to shift forward into the future. For those who are psychoanalytically trained, if what is unfolding in the present moment is only understood as a reflection of past fixations, the present is eclipsed by the past and nuances of change or growth can be missed.

As Daniel Stern (2004) states, "The basic assumption is that *change* is based on lived experience. In and of itself, verbally understanding, explaining, or narrating something is not sufficient to bring about change. There must also be an actual experience, a subjectively lived happening. An event must be *lived*, with feelings and actions taking place in real time, in the real world, with real people in a moment of presentness" (p. 28).

IV   Focusing on the importance of developing techniques and strategies that enhance *right-brain-to-right-brain communication* with our patients (Schore, 2012, 2019) is the fourth way this text addresses unifying theoretical principles and practices. This includes an understanding of the body–brain reaction to trauma, a reflexive activation of the hyper–hypo arousal response system when extreme feelings of fear and/or shame are triggered.

The field of neuroscience has drawn us to reexamine *explicit* and *implicit* aspects of how we process information. Neuroscientific researchers have concluded that the right hemisphere of the brain is linked to *implicit* information processing, whereas the left hemisphere is connected to *explicit* (or more conscious) processing of information. Implicit information processing includes often nonverbal, learned styles of affective response, and learned relational attachment patterns that gets encoded in the first two years of life. These include learned over-compensations to preserve relational connections and habituated defensively based patterns that were meant to preserve homeostatic self-regulation. Attending to the back-and-forth exchange between therapist and client (the serve and return) not only tracks shifts in language and tone of voice, but also the intensity or flattening of affect responses, as well as other nonverbal signals.

Where we have come in our theoretical understanding of early childhood development is that nonverbal cuing, facial expressions, grimacing, and prosity, all reflect the quality of attunement and attachment a child is able to make. Therefore, understanding the client's level of patterning may be much more primitive than how we conducted treatment in the past. Treatment must be designed so as not to recreate nonverbal explosions of micro-aggressions. Right-brain-to-right-brain communication attends to our clients by addressing pre-verbal as well as verbal modes of communication. This, over time, creates a holding environment that can ameliorate failed response patterns in the early parent–child communication patterns.

Beatrice Beebe et al. (2005) state that with regard to the concept of intersubjectivity in the practice of psychodynamic therapies, the primary focus has been on the verbal, explicit mode of communication (p. 2). However, findings from infant researchers (Beebe & Lachmann, 1988; Beebe et al., 2010; Hill, 2015; Lachman & Beebe, 1996; Lyons-Ruth, 1996, 1998, 1999; Lyons-Ruth et al., 2006; Schore, 2012, 2016; Stern, 1985, 1989; Stern et al. 1998; Tronick, 1989, 1998; Tronick et al., 1977) point to the importance of incorporating nonverbal, implicit modes of action-sequences, or procedural knowledge into our understanding of intersubjective, relational practice. In other words, if psychodynamic practice is to be the most useful across a wide range of psychopathologies and attachment injuries, our practice techniques must address both verbal (explicit) and nonverbal (implicit) forms of communication.

V   The fifth unifying principle or theoretical approach is gained through understanding the framework of "Loyalty Contracts." Learned loyalty contracts are the implicit and explicit rules of membership that keep individuals embedded in their family and culture for better or worse. These learned patterns of relationship stem from early attachment styles of interaction that are later replicated through the behaviors and expectations of adult relationships. Understanding a patient's loyalty contract would direct a therapist to examine repeated communication patterns, wishes, longings, expectations, underlying fears, and affective resonance. Learned loyalty contracts are often unconsciously played out in intimate partnerships, in work relationships, and in parenting styles.

The spoken or unarticulated "rules" of The Loyalty Contract that individuals learn in order to preserve relational connection are often in conflict with self-actualizing behaviors. Therefore, a dynamic tension arises internally between wishes and longings for rescue from the old, unfair, or abusive childhood contract and the fear of breaking free and advocating for a healthy self-alternative. This internal tension of the opposites is fueled by the fear of losing membership (covert or overt shunning), coupled with feelings of unworthiness, self-doubt, and/or the belief that no one can be really trusted.

Loyalty contracts are either poorly known by the patient, or they are outside of awareness, or they are accepted as normal. Despite the degree of repetition of dysfunctional patterns and concomitant disappointments, most individuals with varying degrees of attachment disorders seem to have an absence of curiosity or self-reflective capacities to attend to and modify these patterns.

VI   Centering on the power of the therapeutic relationship as a leverage for change is the sixth way this text addresses unifying theoretical principles and practices. How change transpires is dependent on a number of variables, listed as follows:

- The ability to create a safe holding environment
- Adopting a two-person approach to relational dynamics
- Utilizing the unfolding transference and counter-transferential exchanges to repair early attachment injuries
- Facilitating the grieving process as clients let go of unrequited longings from past relational failures
- Ameliorating or neutralizing a person's internalized feelings of shame and unworthiness through the benign witness of the therapist and the reclaiming of one's authentic self.

Largely, this will be played out through transferential enactments with the therapist, where the client can experience a new relational interaction, one that is non-judgmental and encouraging. As stated in our first book (Danielian & Gianotti, 2012).

> Transference *interpersonalizes* the patient's unconscious organizing schemas, schemas which lie at the heart of the patient's character-ological structure. As such, transference constitutes an important cutting edge of therapeutic action, *a live here-and-now enactment* of important material not yet in awareness but edging closer to it. Therefore, as we create foundation stones of understanding, working with transference means working in the subjective present because, first and foremost, this is where the therapeutic dialogue becomes personal.

The mirroring function of the therapeutic relationship comes into play as well. Repeated mirroring over time builds an earned, secure attachment within the parameters of the therapeutic relationship. As the treatment process unfolds, one important dimension of mirroring is the therapist's ability to catch early signs of emerging authenticity, moments in session when the client tentatively begins to test new ways of expressing self in relationship. Using therapeutic mirroring as a technique as well as a therapeutic stance is a way to not only anticipate another person's intentions and resonate with their emotions, but also create right-brain-to-right-brain resonance.

How This Book Is Structured

Each chapter addresses one or several aspects of the theoretical principles and practices described in the previous section of this introduction. A combination of graphic illustrations, case vignettes, and case analyses will be used to illustrate how theoretical principles can be operationalized and applied to practice techniques. A brief description of each chapter follows.

Chapter One introduces two models of psychic organization, one that is defensively driven and the other a healthy, evolving model of the self over the course of the life span. Each model reveals both intrapsychic as well as interpersonal dimensions of the self in relationship. The two visual models of psychic organization are presented with the aim of comparing and contrasting degrees of psychopathology and damage, as well as degrees of evolving resilience and growth. The Four Quadrant Model, introduced in our first two books, illustrates degrees of shame, defensive-overcompensation, and patterns of relational difficulty that patients present to the therapist upon entering treatment. These patterns are found across a wide variety of symptoms and diagnoses. The Healthy Self Model, a new version of the Four Quadrant Model, presents a visual matrix of what the healthy, evolving self looks like throughout the life span.

These two models can be used as a means of considering the various aspects of a patient's presentation, helping the therapist consider presenting problems, emerging strengths, as well as repeated patterns that may be unconscious or hidden from view. By providing this comparison of the two models, therapists can better assess the degree of fragility of their patients as well as discover pockets of resilience and strength that exist along-side of the defensively driven patterns. These models can be used throughout the treatment process as a means of reviewing and tracking progress, healing, and growth.

Chapter Two is devoted to defining and exploring how Learned Loyalty Contracts in childhood manifest as predictive patterns in adulthood. Understanding the wishes and longings as well as fears and defensive re-actions that play out in relationship helps the therapist identify ways to increase conscious awareness of potential blind spots on the part of the patient. By introducing reflective comments and observations, clients are able to bring their own curiosity and insight to begin to change relational interactions and expectations. In addition, how one handles disappointment in relationship will be examined. When dysfunctional relational patterns are conceptualized from the vantage-point of "Learned Loyalty Contracts," therapists are often better equipped to introject questions and increase client curiosity, thus being more successful at interrupting the dysfunctional at-tachment patterns.

Chapter Two further addresses how individual Loyalty Contracts play out within Couples Therapy. Loyalty Contracts in adulthood represent a systemic reenactment of disappointed wishes and longings that are often at the heart of presenting complaints within couples' relationships. This chapter illustrates how communication patterns, hopes, expectations, and disappointments manifest both within and between partners in their intimate relationship as well as within the larger family system. A client example that tracks the treatment over the course of time will be provided to help illustrate how to utilize the Four Quadrant Model within the context of providing couple's therapy. Analysis of the case dialogue will provide practitioners with a tracking system to better assess levels of resilience, defense structures, and degree of flexibility and adaptability.

Chapter Three focuses on case conceptualization and offers a concise way for therapists to take a step back and articulate a big-picture formulation of the dynamic unfolding of a case. The ability to move in and focus on a particular given exchange while simultaneously seeing how the micro-intervention connects to the larger whole of the macro-picture of the patient's presenting issues allows clinicians to pause and assess which parts of the Four-Quadrant Model or dimensions of the psyche may be under-developed or disavowed. This chapter also focuses on points of confusion when the therapeutic frame is too loosely held or when treatment goals and expectations are not clearly articulated from the onset of therapy.

In addition, developing a comprehensive case formulation involves knowing what to look for and what questions to ask. This requires an expansion of the traditional medical model of assessment and dynamic formulation to include questions that measure degrees of affect regulation, quality of attachment, as well as how privilege and marginalization have shaped the patient's sense of self.

Chapter Four addresses specific listening tracking techniques that can be applied to the therapeutic exchange. By slowing down the interactive process, therapists can catch nuances of verbal and nonverbal expression. Furthermore, they can probe to uncover hidden material, and neutralize pockets of shame. Slowing down the process allows for the therapeutic relationship to: increase the intersubjective attunement between therapist and client, facilitate co-regulation of feeling states, and create a new interactive experience in real time over the course of time. Key words or phrases that telegraph potential entry points will be provided through multiple client examples within this chapter. In addition, a graphic model of an iceberg helps to visually illustrate how the moment-to-moment exchange can lead to deeper exploration, one that often reveals hidden affect or repressed historical memory. Various examples of *what to say next* are provided to demonstrate the versatility of this technique.

Chapter Five features the use of entry-points in language to amplify the technique of moment-to-moment tracking. The reader will be provided with case illustrations that highlight a variety of choices that the therapist can make to slow the process down and better track the dynamic exchange. Examples include: tracking the details of the sequence that leads to emotional or behavioral reactivity, using reflection and reframing to help the client identify reflexive thoughts and behavioral patterns, understanding trigger points that lead to shut-down or micro-dissociative moments, and mirroring our clients' responses as a means of allowing them to be seen and validated.

Using therapeutic mirroring as a technique as well as a therapeutic stance is not only a way to anticipate another person's intentions and resonate with their emotions, but also a way to create right-brain-to-right-brain resonance. Repeated mirroring over time builds an earned, secure attachment within the parameters of the therapeutic relationship. As the treatment process unfolds, one important dimension of moment-to-moment tracking through the mirroring response is the therapist's ability to catch early signs of emerging authenticity, moments in session when the client tentatively begins to test new ways of expressing self in relationship. This can take the form of increased insight, curiosity, or self-reflective capacities.

Chapter Six explores how therapists often unwittingly fall victim to colluding with patients around maintaining the split off parts of the psyche. This occurs because either the therapist doesn't recognize or understand the function of defensive splitting, or the therapist mistakes grandiosity as a sign of healthy self-esteem. The defensive function of splitting can be understood as a two-fold process, to keep feelings of shame from coming into conscious awareness, and as a reflexive reaction when unconscious triggers threaten to overwhelm the psyche.

We can better understand the function of splitting through the technique of Part-Whole Analysis. Part-whole analysis is both a theoretical lens from which to apply the Four Quadrant Model and a technique that can be used to reflect back to the client parts of the self that are split off from conscious awareness. This chapter will focus on the technique of "speaking to the splits." Working with the defense mechanism of helps patients move from all or nothing thinking into integrating important aspects of the self into a unified whole. Multiple client examples will be provided to demonstrate ways in which a therapist can wonder about over-and-under reactions to behaviors or events, reflect contradictory statements back to the patient, verbalize unspoken or disavowed wishes and longings, and uncover hidden feelings of vulnerability and shame. It is through integrating split off parts of the self into an ever-evolving whole that healing and recovery from attachment failures can occur.

Chapter Seven illustrates how working with transference and countertransference dynamics within the unfolding therapeutic relationship is a powerful leverage for change in terms of understanding relational enactments and repairing early attachment injuries. All unfinished business from the past is replicated and enacted in present-day relationships; all traumatic events reduce the capacity for curiosity and full functioning. Using these two statements as anchoring points, the discussion of transferential enactments becomes the focus of this chapter. Unconscious, unarticulated, or disavowed material invariably becomes enacted in relationship to others, whether one believes in transference or has been trained in using transference as a leverage of change. Transferential dynamics occur in almost every therapeutic encounter, and yet, many clinicians who have not been trained psycho-dynamically have little if any preparation to anticipate, manage, or invite transferential engagements. Working with transference is one of the most powerful leverages for change, a skill that can be applied across therapeutic disciplines.

It is through the repeated enactments within the unfolding dialogic exchange that transference and counter-transference experiences become the arena in which unrequited longings are grieved, where prohibited anger and disappointment are expressed, and where assumptions around trust and mistrust are worked through. Transferential and counter-transferential reactions will also be explored from the intersubjective theoretical position of co-regulation, and co-creation of the "rhythmic third." Examples will be given as to ways to "invite" transferential exploration as well as to anticipate and palpate the transference before it erupts into damaging, negative transferential enactments. Signs of therapeutic progress can be recognized through the emergence of negative transferential enactments as well. Being able to reflect these authentic aspects of self-expression as they emerge within the treatment hour is a way that newly emerging organizing schemas are built within the psyche. It is also a way that the natural resilience of the psyche can be encouraged and strengthened.

References

Ainsworth, M. D. (1964). Patterns of attachment behavior shown by the infant in interaction with his mother. *Merrill-Palmer Quarterly of Behavior and Development*, *10*, 51–58.

Ainsworth, M. D. S. (1967). *Infancy in Uganda: Infant care and the growth of love*. Johns Hopkins Press.

Ainsworth, M. D. S., & Bell, S. M. (1970). Attachment, exploration, and separation: Illustrated by the behavior of one-year-olds in a strange situation. *Child Development*, *41*, 49–67.

Ainsworth, M. D. S., & Bowlby, J. (1991). An ethological approach to personality development. *American Psychologist*, *46*(4), 331–341.

Alexander, F., & French, T. M. (1946). *Psychoanalytic therapy*. Ronald Press.

Beebe, B., Jaffe, J., Markese, S., Buck, K., Chen, H. Cohen, P., Bahrick, L., Andrews, H., & Felds, S. (2010). The origins of 12-month attachment: A microanalysis of 4-month mother-infant interaction. *Attachment and Human Development*, Jan., *12*(0), 3–141.

Beebe, B., Knoblauch, S., Rustin, J., & Sorter, D. (2005). *Forms of intersubjectivity in infant research and adult treatment*. Other Press.

Beebe, B., & Lachmann, F. (1988). The contribution of mother-infant mutual influence to the origins of self – and object representations. *Psychoanalytic Psychology 5*(4), 305–337.

Bowlby, J. (1951). Maternal care and mental health (2nd Ed.). *World Health Organization. Monograph*, *3*, 355–534.

Bowlby, J. (1958). The nature of the child's tie to his mother. *International Journal of PsychoAnalysis*, *39*, 1–23.

Cooper, S. H. (2010). *A disturbance in the field: Essays in transference-countertransference engagement*. Routledge.

Cyr, C., Euser E. M., Bakermans-Kranenburg, M. J., & Van Ijzendoorn, M. H. (2010). Attachment security and disorganization in maltreating and high-risk families: A series of meta-analyses. *Development and Psychopathology, Winter*, *22*(1), 87–108.

Danielian, J., & Gianotti, P. (2012). *Listening with purpose: Entry points into shame and narcissistic vulnerability*. Routledge.

Dutra L., Bureau J. F., Holmes B., Lyubchik A., & Lyons-Ruth, K. (2009). Quality of early care and childhood trauma: A prospective study of developmental pathways to dissociation. *Journal of Nervous and Mental Disease*, *197*(6), 383–390.

Ferenczi, S. (1919). Contra-indications to the "active" psycho-analytical technique. In J. Rickman (Ed.) & J. Suttie (Trans.), *Further contributions to the theory and technique of psycho-analysis*, (pp. 189–197). Boni and Liveright.

Ferenczi, S., & Rank. O. (1925). *The development of psycho-analysis* (C. Newton, Trans.). Nervous and Mental Disease Publishing.

Frank, R., & LaBarre, F. (2010). *The first year and the rest of your life: Movement, development, and psychotherapeutic change*. Routledge.

Gianotti, P., & Danielian, J. (2017). *Uncovering the resilient core: A workbook on the treatment of narcissistic defenses, shame, and emerging authenticity*. Routledge.

Goldfried, M. R. (Ed.) (1982). *Converging themes in psychotherapy: Trends in psychodynamic, humanistic, and behavioral practice*. New York: Springer.

Goldfried, M. R. (2019). Obtaining consensus in psychotherapy: What holds us back? *American Psychologist*, *74*(4), 484–496.

Hazanov, V. (2019). *Fear of doing nothing: Notes of a young therapist*. Aeon Books.

Hill, D. (2015). *Affect regulation theory: A clinical model*. W. W. Norton & Co.

Horney, K. (1950). *Neurosis and human growth: The struggle toward self-realization*. Norton.

Lachmann, F., & Beebe, B. (1996). Three principles of salience in the organization of the patient-analyst interaction. *Psychoanalytic Psychology* *13*(1), 1–22.

Lyons-Ruth, K. (1996). Attachment relationships among children with aggressive behavior problems: the role of disorganized early attachment patterns. *Journal of Consulting and Clinical Psychology*, *64*(1), 32–40.

Lyons-Ruth, K. (1998). Implicit relational knowing: Its role in development and psychoanalytic treatment. *Infant Mental Health Journal*, *19*(3), 282–291.

Lyon-Ruth, K. (1999). The two-person unconscious: Intersubjective dialogue, enactive relational representation, and the emergence of new forms of relational organization. *Psychoanalytic Inquiry*, *19*(4), 576–617.

Lyons-Ruth, K., Dutra, L., Schuder, M., & Banchi, L. (2006). From infant attachment disorganization to adult dissociation: Relational adaptations for traumatic experiences. *Psychiatric Clinics of North America*, *29*(1) 63–86.

Mitchell, S. A. (1993). *Hope and dread in psychoanalysis*. Harper Collins.

Ogawa, J., Sroufe, L. A., & Weinfield, N. S. (1997). Development and the fragmented self: A longitudinal study of dissociate symptomatology in a non-clinical sample. *Development and Psychopathology*, *9*(4), 855–879.

Pally, R. (1998). Emotional processing: The mind-body connection. *International Journal of Psychoanalysis. Psychoanalytic Inquiry*, *21*, 71–93.

Pally, R. (2000). *The mind-brain relationship*. Other Press.

Schore, A. N. (2012). *The science of the art of psychotherapy*. W. W. Norton & Company.

Schore, A. N. (2016). *Affect regulation and the origin of the self: The neurobiology of emotional development*. Psychology Press and Routledge Classic Editions.

Schore, A. N. (2019). *Right brain psychotherapy*. W. W. Norton & Company.

Stern, D. (1985). *The interpersonal world of the infant*. Basic Books.

Stern, D. (1989). The representation of relational patterns: Developmental considerations. In A. Sameroff and R. Emde (Eds), *Relationship disturbances in early childhood: A developmental approach*, (pp. 52–69). Basic Books.

Stern, D. (2004). *The present moment in psychotherapy and everyday life*. W. W. Norton & Company.

Stern D., Sander, L., Nahum, J., Harrison, A. M., Lyons-Ruth, K., Morgan, A. C., Bruschweiler-Stern, N., & Tronick, E. Z. (1998). Non-interpretive mechanisms in psychoanalytic therapy. *International Journal of Psychoanalysis*, *79*(5), 903–921.

Stone, L. (1961). *The psychanalytic situation: An examination of its development and essential nature*. International Universities Press, Inc.

Tronick, E. (1989). Emotions and emotional communication in infants. *American Psychologist*, *44*(2), 112–119.

Tronick, E. Z. (1998). Dyadically expanded states of consciousness and the process of therapeutic change. *Infant Mental Health Journal 19*(3), 290–299.

Tronick, E., Als, H., & Adamson, L. (1977). Structure of early face-to-face communicative interactions. In M. Bullowa (Ed), *Before speech* (pp. 349–372). Cambridge University Press.

1 Creating a Three-Dimensional Matrix of the Psyche: Contrasting Two Roadmaps of Relational Development

Introduction

Imagine, if you will, a healthy, intact human being. Does such a person exist, and if so, can we agree upon what he or she looks like? What are the dimensions of self and self-in-relationship that we would use to assess the quality of health, spontaneity, authenticity, whole-heartedness, ambition, resilience, and personal growth throughout the life span? As therapists we are in the business of healing and transformation, of repairing psychic injuries that accumulate as a result of insecure attachment bonds, trauma, cultural inequity, isolation, and racism. Yet, our approach to treating psychological injuries vary according to one's theoretical orientation and training in combination with the needs, goals, and resources of our clients. This creates a complicated picture of precisely how to proceed with treatment, one in which therapists have argued over for more than a century.

In an attempt to create unifying principles around factors that contribute to health and psychic disease, this chapter presents two visual graphics of psychic development. One graphic describes individuals who were afforded the opportunity to thrive in a safe, secure, and loving environment, and the other describes individuals who suffered from varying degrees of trauma, deprivation, and/or insecurity in childhood. The outcome of a healthy upbringing allows for the unique qualities of the self to be supported in the context of providing fair and consistent rules of relational engagement that foster a sense of mutuality, where respect for self and other are treated equally. The outcome of an upbringing where the unique qualities of one's self had to be sacrificed in order to preserve a precarious attachment with fragile, disorganized, or narcissistic care-givers results in varying degrees of insecurity, affect dysregulation, traumatically induced neurological and physiologically embedded injury, and acquired defense structures that attempt to compensate for these losses and limitations.

What do these two pictures of psychic development look like as individuals evolve throughout the life span? This chapter presents two models that can be used as assessment tools when evaluating the spectrum of health

DOI: 10.4324/9781003120278-2

and illness. Regardless of one's theoretical training and expertise, these models provide therapists with a template that illuminates factors that comprise defense structures, psychic stability, degrees of self-care, and the dimensions and quality of interpersonal relationships.

Measures that Depict Health, Fragility, and Psychic Stability

Identifying qualities that contribute to mental/emotional health is not a new concept to the field of psychology. There are numerous theories as well as lists of attributes that determine psychological health (Fredrickson & Losada, 2005; Markstrom & Marshall, 2006; Metz, 1961; Peterson, Park, & Seligman, 2004; Seligman, 2004; Vallerand et al., 2003.) A list of quality that measure aspects of psychological health, taken from the *Psychodynamic Diagnostic Manual* include a number of specific capacities such as:

- self-regulation, attention and learning,
- intimacy and mutuality in relationships,
- differentiation & integration,
- self-reflection,
- constructing and applying internal standards of morality,
- assimilating new learning,
- creativity and curiosity.

Adler (1930); Allport (1943, 1950); Bellak and Sheehy (1976); Erickson (1950); and Fairbairn (1952) all speak of ego strengths that contribute to stability and well-being. These include measures of a person's temperament, motivation, and psychological mindedness, that increase an individual's personal and social competence as well as contributing to psychic stability in times of stress. In addition, ego strengths such as self-efficacy, intelligence, and cognitive flexibility are closely related to openness and creativity, and successfully adapting to external stimuli. Psychological flexibility, which is measured by the capacity to tolerate certain degrees of distress while maintaining psychic equilibrium is a critical measure of psychic resilience (Hayes et al., 1996; Kashdan & Rottenberg, 2010). In general ego capacities reflect the quality of one's internal experience as measured by level of confidence and self-regard, one's affective experience, and the quality of expression, and communication. Deficiencies in any of these areas result in greater difficulty managing life's challenges (Gfellner & Cordoba, 2017; Hartmann, 1958; Kagle & Levay, 1977).

In my first two books, written with co-author, Jack Danielian, we provided a visual matrix of patients who present with varying degrees of psychic injury. We entitled this graphic the Four Quadrant Model, a model that simultaneously captures a picture of intrapsychic, relational, systemic, and socio-cultural aspects of an individual. Regardless of symptom presentation or diagnosis, this model enabled therapists to better understand the interaction between shame, self-stability, fears, expectations, and longings for interpersonal connection. It measured how individuals respond to disappointment, and it provided therapists a means to assess degrees of defensive over-compensation that individuals use in an attempt to keep feelings of shame and inadequacy from breaking into conscious awareness.

Since the development of the Four Quadrant Model and the publication of our first two books, we began using this model as a teaching tool in our advanced training programs, public lectures, and continuing education seminars. We soon discovered that clinicians were often confused about the sometimes-fine-line between healthy self-esteem and pathological over-compensation that masqueraded as success in the outside world. This confusion meant that therapists often misjudged the toll that defensive over-compensations took on their patients over time.

Defensive solutions that attempt to mask feelings of inadequacy are ultimately unsustainable because the drive to continually prove self-worth will deplete a person's energy over time. Defensively based behavioral patterns create a vicious cycle in that they never permanently ameliorate one's core sense of underlying shame. These never-ending cyclic patterns of overcompensation eventually lead to symptomatic break-through, or in cases of severe trauma or deprivation, they can lead to psychic fragmentation. The toll on the psyche may be subtle at first, and therefore difficult to recognize, but over time these patterns drain vitality, resulting in increased rigidity, resignation, and/or resentment.

The Healthy Self-Actualizing Model presented for the first time in this book was created to illustrate specific attributes and measures of healthy development throughout the life span. This model is meant to serve as a companion piece to the Four Quadrant Model to help practitioners more easily recognize how healthy behaviors fuel and invigorate psychic vitality rather than drain psychic energy. The Healthy Self-Actualizing Model, with a similar graphic design as the Four Quadrant Model, presents a matrix that highlights degrees of evolving resilience and growth. The identified qualities in each quadrant can be used as a means of placing the various aspects of a patient's presentation in a context, where defense structures are weighed along-side a patient's strengths and resilience. Using the two models together can also help therapists recognize when defensive patterns begin to give way to emerging signs of growth throughout the treatment process.

Therapists can draw upon these models as a diagnostic tool, in assessing levels of symptom severity, setting treatment goals, as well as increasing proficiency around treatment interventions throughout the course of therapy. We have found that by providing a comparison of the two models, therapists can better assess the degree of fragility and shame sensitivity as well as discover pockets of resilience and strength that exist along-side of the defensively driven patterns. In that regard the two models can be used *throughout* the treatment process as a means of reviewing and tracking therapeutic progress.

Personal clinical styles often become more routinized over time. The longer we work with a patient and hear repeated stories, there is a drift toward assuming we know what the patient is saying, which may result in missing nuances of communication or other important parts of the client's narrative. Those parts of the relational dynamic that remain under-attended or minimized are often aspects of the patient's psyche that are either consciously hidden, or they are unconsciously enacted within the therapeutic relationship. Clinical blind spots, left unattended, often reveal a shared, intersubjective dynamic that has developed between client and therapist. More often than not, these blind spots eventually create a stalemate in the treatment and result in some degree of frustration on the part of both parties.

What the Four Quadrant Model and Healthy Self-Actualization Model can provide is a type of a safety net, a reference point where clinicians can check-in with themselves or confer with colleagues when moments of therapeutic impasse occur. Using the Four Quadrant Model as a reference point, clinicians often discover areas of the psyche that may have received little attention in terms of therapeutic inquiry. For example, some clinicians may focus more on relational dynamics while under attending to intrapsychic conflicts. Others attend exclusively to symptom reduction, where others work to change negative cognitions. Using the Healthy Self-Actualizing model allows us to more easily recognize the areas of strength that the patient has used to master challenges and attain a sense of authentic accomplishment. Using these two models as a dual reference point during the course of treatment can assist in keeping the complexity of therapeutic attention in the forefront, attending to both areas of defensive constraint as well as areas of health and resilience.

The Structural Design of the Two Models

Some of the content presented in the next section of this chapter has been drawn for our first two publications. The Four Quadrant Model will be reviewed and explained in this chapter. However, for a more detailed description, please refer to Chapter Two, pages 32–61 of *Listening with Purpose: Entry Points into Shame and Narcissistic Vulnerability,* and Chapter Four, pages 57–94 of *Uncovering the Resilient Core: A Workbook on the Treatment of Narcissistic Defenses, Shame, and Emerging Authenticity.*

The structural design of the two models is broken up into four different quadrants (Figure 1.1), each representing its own psychic function. Although both graphic models separate these components of the self into four different quadrants, when viewed as a whole, the model is meant to capture a dynamic composite of interconnected parts that are either integrated or split off from one another. Each of the four quadrants in both models maintain varying degrees of conscious awareness/attention at any given time, depending on both external and internal triggers.

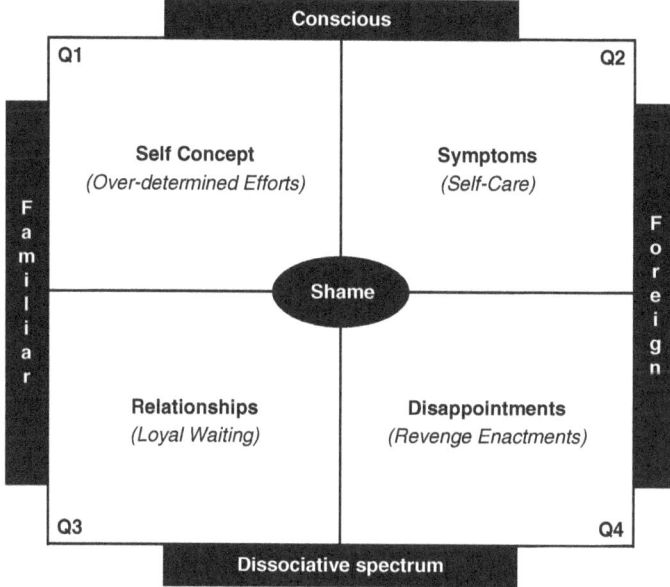

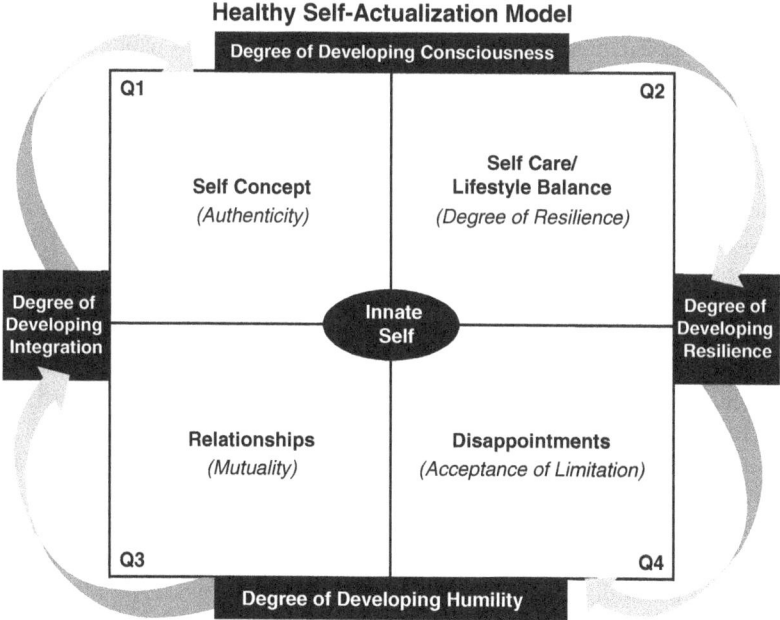

Figure 1.1 Two Model Comparison.

The Four Quadrant Model, which is on the top, offers a picture that captures the defensively based character organization of individuals who suffered from early attachment failures. When trauma or neglect impact the degree of safety and security in childhood, conditions that are necessary for the developing self to thrive, the formation of a secure attachment fails to occur. As a result, feelings of confusion, fear, and a core sense of unworthiness become internalized, producing defensively based behaviors and beliefs that then become used in an attempt to over-compensate for feelings of inadequacy through repeatedly trying to prove self-worth. This diagram presents a structural map or *organizing schema*, that represents a person's core beliefs about self as well as relational expectations of others.

Insecure attachments produce personality structures that are best understood on a continuum of defensively based rigidity or flexibility. In the Four Quadrant Model the thoughts, values, behaviors, beliefs, and expectation of self and others illustrate some degree of over-determination and compulsivity. These personality styles often display varying degrees of reactivity, impulsivity, under or over-attention to self-care, and acts of retaliation that surface when longings, wishes, and personal ambitions are thwarted. Because the Four Quadrant Model illustrates a character structure that is defensively driven, there is an overall lack of integration *between* each of the quadrants as well. Thus, capacities such as self-reflection, lifestyle balance, and to learn from one's mistakes are inhibited.

Although the individual's over-determined efforts are aimed at maintaining hope, a positive sense of self, and affective stability, the cost of this type of character organization is that the capacity to change and grow throughout the lifespan is compromised. Thus, we see a personality that is fraught with repeating dysfunctional patterns. These patterns attempt to serve the function of maintaining the over-idealized belief in perfectionism, both in the self as well as the wish for a perfectly attuned partner. Unfortunately, these efforts are in opposition to the emergence of authentic self-expression. They also present a challenge to the real work of psychotherapy, where feelings of shame and the grieving past attachment failures must be confronted and metabolized.

The Healthy Self-Actualizing Model assumes that the innate self was allowed to develop with relatively little interference throughout the life span. Any challenges to the emergence of the authentic self were able to be resolved, either by negotiating one's needs with caregivers toward a satisfactory resolution or through the course of a successful therapeutic encounter. Therefore, the distinction between conscious vs. dissociative process (as shown in the Four Quadrant Model) is replaced with circular arrows that surround each of the quadrants, depicting on-going growth with regard to capacities that reflect, a). increasing consciousness, b). resilience, c). humility, and d). integration. Symptoms are replaced with lifestyle balance that helps regulate external and internal demands on the psyche. Personal growth continues throughout the life cycle without having the losses or disappointments of life turn the individual into someone with regret, bitterness, or stagnation.

Both models represent a schematic that captures how people experience themselves in relation to others, as well as what they expect, how they manage complicated feeling states, and how they negotiate strategies for living. Each of these models represent an organizing schematic that illuminates the internal processes of the personality, one that is generative, and one that is defensively driven. A brief definition of what each quadrant represents is as follows.

- Quadrant One of both models represents the consciously held beliefs, values, motivations, and strivings of the self as a unique individual.
- Quadrant Two represents lifestyle balance, or lack thereof, the result of which is either the maintenance of physical, psychological, and spiritual vitality in the Healthy Self-Actualization Model, or the inattention or diminishment of self-care that results in symptomatic break-through in the Four Quadrant Model.
- Quadrant Three represents how the individual relates to others within the context of family, workplace, and intimate relationships.
- Quadrant Four represents how the individual responds to disappointment, either with oneself or with others.

In the Model representing Healthy Self-Actualization, the four quadrants or four aspects of the self are relatively well-integrated and in communication with each other. Personal strivings and ambitions come from a sense of fulfilling one's purpose, giving back to the world, and the desire for personal growth throughout the life span. When healthy individuals experience a conflict, a challenge, a growth opportunity, a disappointment, or an unexpected loss, they are able to exhibit:

- the *capacity for self-reflection,*
- a *desire to ask for help and a willingness to receive help,*
- *an ability to admit mistakes,*
- *an ability to apologize,*
- *and to eventually forgive self or others for wrong doings.*

Spontaneity, humility, playfulness, a spirit of whole-heartedness, creativity, curiosity, and compassion are aspects of a healthy, evolving self.

The Four Quadrant Model represents a picture of individuals who suffered from trauma, deprivation, or varying degrees of insecure attachment, and because of this the four quadrants are generally not well integrated. Personal strivings and ambitions found in Quadrant One are often overdetermined and compulsively driven in an attempt to prove self-worth, therefore the idea of self-care is seen as unimportant. Relationships with others are either over-idealized or met with mistrust. Reaction to disappointment often triggers feelings of shame and a consequent response of retaliation or self-punishment, rather than drawing upon self-reflective capacities to help gain perspective and learn from mistakes. All quadrants represented in the Four Quadrant Model reflect some degree of compulsivity, imbalance, or unconscious repetition of self-defeating patterns, all of which are an outcome of varying degrees of attachment failures in childhood.

Attachment failures predictably will result in adults who possess an under-developed sense of self, an inability to self-soothe, and a mistrust that others will be of support. Because safety, security, and the attendant development of neuronal pathways were compromised in childhood, these individuals reflexively learn to do whatever it would take to preserve a tenuous sense of attachment to parental figures. This often meant sacrificing key components of the authentic self in order to survive. It also meant learning to develop strategies, beliefs, and behaviors to hide or compensate for an internalized sense of shame and unworthiness that became internalized and deeply held within the core sense of who they are. Therefore, these individuals often exhibit behaviors and beliefs that are rigidly held and compulsively over-determined in order that they can prove their sense of worthiness to others or make sure that no one takes advantage of them.

A More Detailed Description of the Models

The first model, The Four Quadrant Model (Figure 1.2), represents a picture of individuals who developed a defensively based organizing structure that functions in an attempt to maintain a homeostatic balance in the service of regulating feeling states, and preserving a positive self-image. Notice that the graphic model places shame at the center, connecting all four quadrants, because the responses contained within each of the quadrants were defensively created, consciously and/or unconsciously, in an attempt to keep feelings of shame outside of conscious awareness.

The left side of the diagram represents feelings, beliefs, aspirations, and desires that are identified by the individual as acceptable, congruent, or they are at least tolerated in terms of self-identity. Quadrant One and Quadrant Three are placed on the left side of the diagram because they are experienced as relatively comfortable/familiar and therefore are more easily incorporated into the conscious experience of self. Although there are parts of both the individual (Q1) and relational aspects of the self (Q3) that fall outside of conscious awareness, the parts that *are* consciously acknowledged are not perceived as threatening or foreign. Rather they are absorbed into a congruent sense of "This is who I am."

The right side of the diagram represents feeling states or impulses that feel uncomfortable and/or foreign to one's sense of self. Quadrant Two and Quadrant Four are placed on the right side of the diagram because the feelings or impulses that arise from these two quadrants contain a

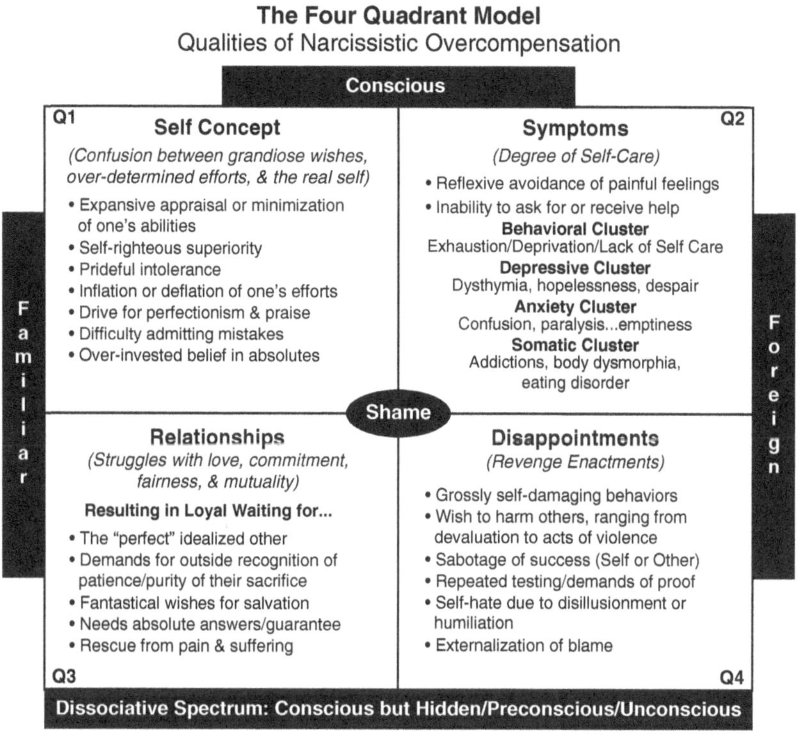

The Four Quadrant Model
Qualities of Narcissistic Overcompensation

Figure 1.2 The Four Quadrant Model.

destructive or threatening element; therefore, they cannot be easily contained or absorbed into one's sense of self. When aspects of Quadrants Two or Four begin to break into conscious awareness, there is a reflexive impulse to shut down or minimize feeling states and the resulting impulses that may arise. If minimization fails to reestablish a homeostatic balance of affect regulation or an improved sense of self-worth, then increased discomfort or decompensation is likely to occur.

You will also notice that at the bottom of Quadrant Three and Quadrant Four (the descriptor that identifies the *Dissociative Spectrum*) is a representation of the range of awareness from conscious to unconsciousness. Consciousness is fluid and is subject to macro and micro breaks in awareness based on external triggers or dysregulated internal emotional states. Paul Wachtel (2008) states that consciousness is not fixed, and he describes the fluid quality of consciousness as a state of *knowing and not knowing* at the same time. For example, we can know something intellectually but not feel the emotional impact. We can remember that a spouse abused us last week, but we still believe things will be different this time. We can know that walking down a dark alley at night is dangerous, but we can also minimize this danger because we feel lucky, invincible, or get a thrill from walking too close to the edge. Or we can utter a disparaging remark about someone and justify it by saying the person deserved it, thus preserving our own positive self-image.

The placement of the dissociative spectrum underneath Quadrants Three and Four is meant to highlight the fact that these two quadrants generally contain a greater degree of disavowed or unacknowledged affect; more is hidden from self or others in terms of the residue of primitive impulses, fears, and longings. The examples in the above paragraph illustrating the dissociative spectrum – the knowing and not knowing of awareness – represent parts of the self that are in conflict with other parts and have not been fully integrated into one's conscious narrative. Therefore, important aspects of self, that are *active,* as evidenced by repeated patterns of enactment, remain largely outside of conscious awareness. They have not been metabolized into the narrative of *this is who I am.* It is the slow methodical process of psychotherapy that allows for the integration of these split-off aspects of the self.

As you study the model, notice that each quadrant contains beliefs or behaviors that are either over-determined or under-attended. In that regard each of the quadrants contain elements that are poorly known or disavowed. Therefore, there is some degree of splitting that is occurring in each of the four quadrants. Depending on the degree of defensive rigidity, there may be a *quality of impenetrability* to the individual's psychic make-up, where aspects of reality or "fact-checking" are often minimized, even denied, in order to preserve a fragile sense of psychic stability. Any disagreement, any piece of information that runs counter to what the individual wishes to believe may run the risk of threatening the homeostatic balance. Degrees of impenetrability vs receptivity can be viewed on a continuum as well, where higher degrees of receptivity are predictive of a more positive therapeutic outcome, and greater degrees of impenetrability require a more careful approach to the therapeutic process.

Below is a description of each of the quadrants and the response patterns when the homeostatic balance is threatened.

- In Quadrant One, psychic stability is threatened if efforts around achievement or one's values and beliefs are challenged or threatened. A **cardinal feature of Quadrant One is the desire and belief that one can achieve perfectionism**. Over-determined efforts to achieve the idealized fantasy of perfection helps to bolster the individual's sense of competence while preventing core feelings of inadequacy from collapsing personal initiative.
- In Quadrant Two, psychic stability is threatened when symptoms begin to emerge. The infallible, idealized sense of self in Quadrant One begins to break down when symptoms emerge. This in turn engages feelings of shame that threaten to enter consciousness, which

simultaneously activates Quadrant Four in terms of lashing out against self or others. A *cardinal feature of Quadrant Two is the wish to "fix" the problematic symptoms without altering lifestyle,* **beliefs, or over-idealized ambitions**.

- In Quadrant Three, psychic stability is threatened when relational longings are disappointed, or when intimate partners or other idealized figures appear to fall short in the person's eyes. A *cardinal feature of Quadrant Three reflects an absence of mutuality as well as unrealistic expectations of others.* Relational longings and expectations of others are in the service of ameliorating past attachment failures.

- In Quadrant Four, psychic stability is threatened by disappointment in either the interpersonal arena or failed individual pursuits. A *cardinal feature of Quadrant Four is the desire to retaliate against others or punish the self* around disappointed expectations.

You can see how the Four Quadrant matrix is a tightly woven construction of interconnecting parts. When any one quadrant is activated by the disappointment of idealized longings or personal aspirations, it threatens to bring feelings of shame to the surface, thus, destabilizing the defense structure. Think about the relationship between the quadrants as a fulcrum – when someone feels that their sense of self is injured (Q1), or relational disappointment occurs (Q3), it will activate (Q4) in one of two ways – turning against the self or the other. If one turns against self, the function of this behavior is to reactivate the over-idealized wish for perfection. "I failed; therefore, I deserve to feel shame, and if I punish myself enough, I'll be able to do it better next time." If the person lashes out against others, this avoids the experience of personal shame. "You hurt me, and now I'm justified in trying to make you feel worse." Thus, the system is rebalanced by making the "other", rather than the self, the target of shame.

Both retaliatory strategies work for a brief period of time, until another disappointment happens. Then, the defensively based homeostatic balance becomes threatened once again, and more energy, more effort is required to reestablish psychic equilibrium. This is why defensive solutions aren't effective in the long run. They take too much energy to maintain, and people get weary, resulting in symptom break-through. Over time if these patterns are left unattended, symptoms generally get worse. Because defensively based organizing schemas are in the service of preventing shame from coming into conscious awareness, therefore shame cannot be processed so that the negative feelings and beliefs can be understood, metabolized, and resolved. Rather, shame is seen as an enemy, something to fight against rather than understood.

Thus, defensive solutions perpetuate a "vicious cycle", where a new goal, a new effort, a new partner is believed to provide rescue of the self from suffering or to prove once and for all the person's worthiness. This pattern of behavior is unsustainable because the core attachment injuries are never fully understood. When grief over past pain and maltreatment is never allowed to be fully felt or acknowledged, release and transformation are not able to occur. Thus, the vicious cycle continues.

The Health Self-Actualizing Model

In the next section we will examine the Healthy Self-Actualizing Model. Although no one experiences a perfectly loving, non–injurious childhood, this diagram is designed to illustrate how the resolution of minor to moderate injuries can, in fact, produce an intact, healthy, self-actualizing human being. Everyone has experienced some struggle or conflict in life that created a hindrance to authentic self-emergence; yet, despite pain and setbacks, for many individuals it is possible to pursue self-actualization, discover a sense of purpose, and achieve and maintain healthy, loving relationships.

Healthy narcissism in adulthood is a misnomer. A little bit of narcissism is *not* a good thing. Healing narcissistic injury is quite possible, however, this is dependent upon:

- the extent of early damage,
- the degree of external support and opportunity,
- and the quality of therapeutic interaction and other healthy, inspiring relational encounters.

The process of healthy self-actualization is never without struggle and an-xiety, even for individuals who move through the developmental phases relatively intact. As Freud (1905, 1926) reminded us, in order for a child to move forward into each new developmental phase (from symbiosis through the gradual steps of separation-individuation), just the right amount of an-xiety is necessary to propel forward development. Too much anxiety, and the child becomes overwhelmed, unable to move forward. Too little anxiety and the comfort and reliance on caregivers maintains a state of dependence and passivity. Object relations theorists and ego psychologists (Bion, 1962, 1963; Erickson, 1950; Fairbairn, 1952; Guntrip, 1971; Hartmann et al., 1964; Klein, 1952, Klein & Riviere, 1964; Mahler et al., 1975; Mitchell, 1993, 1997, Mitchell & Black, 1995; Rapaport, 1950; Winnicott, 1951, 1958, 1960) frame forward developmental movement as the ability to resolve or work through relational difficulties and struggles through the corrective emotional experience of a real relationship. If developmental milestones were arrested due to insecure attachment with parental figures, a reparative ex-perience could occur as an outcome of the patient and therapist relationship. This working through includes confronting issues around intimacy, control, loss, trust, and dependency/autonomy. These corrective experiences can occur outside of the context of therapy as well, in the form of a reliable relative, teacher, mentor, peer support group.

In addition, part of healthy growth and development inevitably involves a continual process of relinquishing over-idealized fantasies and over-reliance on attachment figures, whether that be parental figures, mentors, spiritual advisors, or any person in a position of reverence or leadership. A *fall from grace* of these important figures invariably happens when we begin to see the idealized person's shortcomings and experience varying degrees of disappointment. If the idealized attachment figure disappoints us in minimal ways, the grieving of the loss of the ideal allows us to adjust to a more realistic version of who the individual is while still maintaining a sense of appreciation and respect. If we experience a shattering of the idealization due to an egregious disappointment such as betrayal or deceit, the fall from grace is much more painful and injurious, and it can have a lasting effect on our ability to trust in the future.

Grieving the loss of the idealized object includes letting go of wishes and longings based on idealized fantasies of *what could be or could have been*. This grieving process admittedly does take a bit of the mystery and magic out of life. However, if the grieving process occurs in the presence of a secure connection with a trusted other, the wished-for mystery and magic can be exchanged for a more grounded perspective, increased personal efficacy, increased self-confidence, and increased humility, coupled with an ability to move into a fuller and more complete actualization of one's authentic, innate self.

The de-idealization process, where self-object internalizations shift toward a more realistic view of others (Goldberg & Stepansky, 1984; Kohut, 1971, 1977; Ornstein, 1978) has a concomitant effect of altering one's views of the self as well. The grieving of the ideal allows for the blossoming of a more realistic picture of who we are. We can grow in our ability to internalize a greater appreciation of our value. In addition, our goals and aspirations often come into clearer alignment. It also makes room for a more realistic picture of what we can expect from our interpersonal relationships moving forward. Mastering fears of isolation, memory traces of abandonment, along with the innate desire to engage in the world through the reliance on our own resources are primary task of normal development. If avoided, the natural, on-going adult developmental process begins to slow down or shut down, as measured by a slowing down of curiosity, optimism, personal transformation, and physical vitality.

External factors such as war, senseless cruelty, tragic loss, systemic racism or classism, or physical illness certainly are challenges to ongoing growth and optimism throughout the life span. Yet, healthier individuals weather these storms with a sense of hope while their social connections remain intact. The motivation for creating a model that illustrates what healthy self-actualization can look like is important because it reminds clinicians of what is possible in terms of growth throughout the life span. The Healthy Self-Actualizing Model, provided below, is a realistic picture of attributes, capacities, beliefs, and behaviors that reflect a reinforcing feedback loop that is self-sustaining. This sustainability is dependent on the reliance and support of others as well as personal responsibility and proactivity around ongoing engagement in life.

Healthy Self–Actualizing Model

The diagram below shows what a self that is *not* narcissistically driven might look like. Each of the quadrants reflect achievable, realistic attributes and behaviors. Although most of these qualities have to be learned and earned, it does illustrate that healing, growth, and maintaining vitality throughout the life span is achievable.

You will notice a similarity in design of the Healthy Self-Sustaining Model (Figure 1.3) and the Four Quadrant Model. Each of the four quadrants in both models contain similar categories that represent similar psychic functions. However, in the place of symptoms, you will find Self-Care and Lifestyle Balance. In place of over-determined efforts to

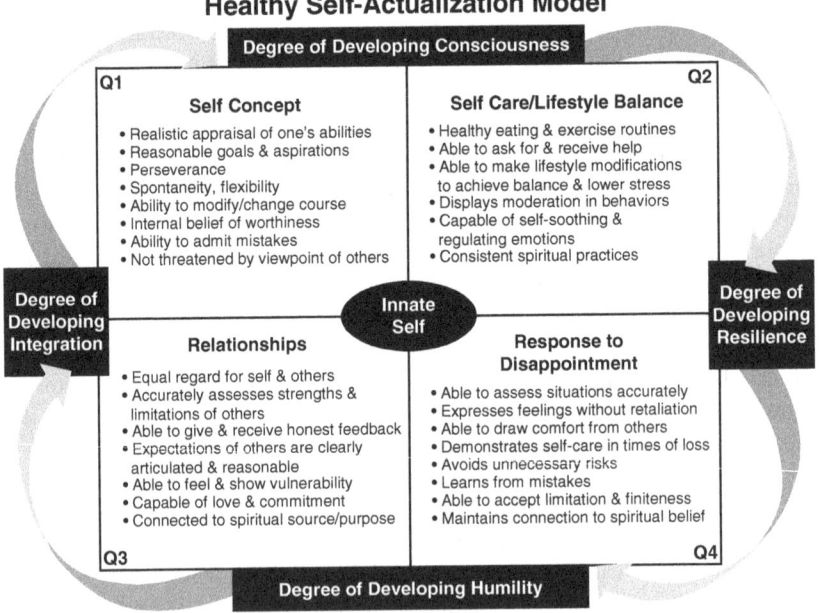

Figure 1.3 Healthy Self-Actualization Model.

avoid feelings of shame, the individual is motivated by an internal sense of authentic self-acceptance.

The outer edges of the model represent an evolving cyclical loop of developing degrees of consciousness, resilience, humility, and integration. The descriptors of comfort and discomfort, conscious and dissociate spectrum found in the Four Quadrant Model are replaced with the four categories contained within the revolving arrows. They reflect the receptivity and interaction between external and internal forces that are at play on the system. The arrows symbolize that the growth process is never complete. Learning and refinement continue well into old age.

Rather than shame being placed in the center of the diagram, the innate self is what connect all four quadrants together. The innate self is what fuels motivation and attributes as well as the functions that are contained within each quadrant. The systemic nature of the model illustrates how each quadrant sustains and informs the development of the others. An obvious difference in the Healthy Self-Actualizing Model is that defensive over-determination is supplanted with a realistic appraisal of achievement, realistic expectations of self and other, an ability to grieve, and a gentle, self-reflective approach to handling disappointment and learning from mistakes. There is a quality of acceptance rather than resistance around the inevitability of the very real limitations of life – such as, the limitation of time, energy, capacity, choice, opportunity, and aging. In no way is the Healthy Self-Actualizing Model meant to reflect any form of resignation or defeat. It simply is a picture of mature, healthy adulthood.

If you view both diagrams side-by-side (Figures 1.4 and 1.5), you can more clearly see how learned defense structures interfere with growth and development across the life span. Efforts to avoid shame interfere with or mask the innate self's development and unique capacities and contributions. The core, innate self is a construct that is meant to capture what it means to be human. It is a construct that relies on the assumption that resilience is an innate part of the true self. So, when you remove the defensive over-compensations of the false self that had been a hinderance to authentic self-emergence, the innate self can emerge.

One of the components that was added to the Healthy Self-Actualizing Model, not contained in the Four Quadrant Model, is the element of *spirituality*. As we have begun to incorporate spiritual techniques such as mindfulness meditation and yoga and other practices aimed at helping to recover from psychological trauma, the element of spirituality was added to the model. These techniques or spiritual disciplines contribute to lifestyle balance, neuropsychological healing, and the sense of "who I am". It also increases the capacity for and the desire to move toward forgiveness and to seek some form of communion with that which is larger than the self.

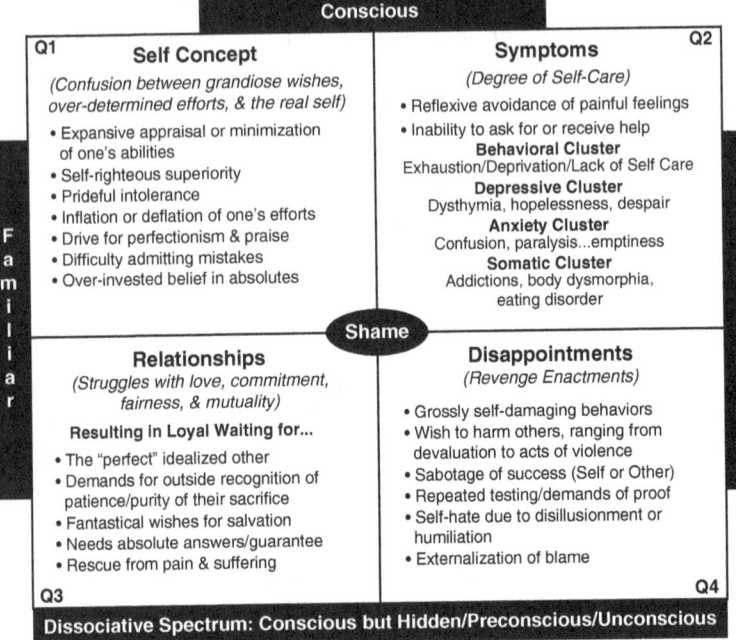

Figure 1.4 The Four Quadrant Model.

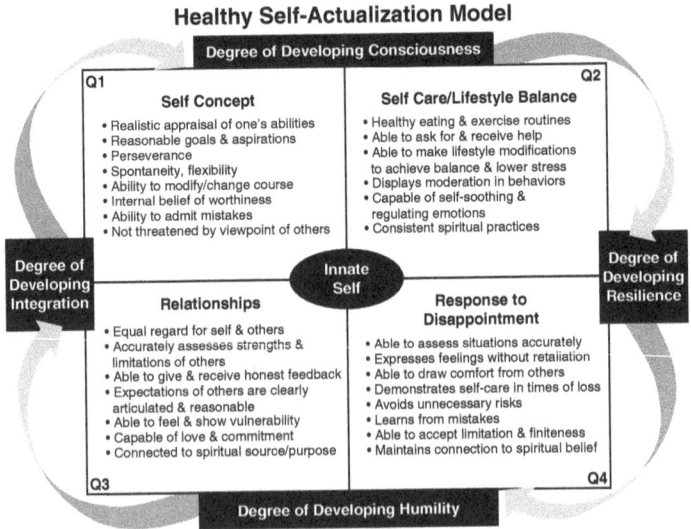

Figure 1.5 Healthy Self-Actualization Model.

How to Use the Two Models in Assessment and the Treatment Process

As clinicians it is our job to measure the *severity* of symptom presentation, the *degree* of pathology and the underlying *intensity* of affect that our patients are defending against. This in turn will determine the *pace* in which the therapeutic process unfolds. It also will determine the *goals* of treatment and the *approach* we will take to help the patient achieve affect regulation and stability, as well as helping them uncover and repair old attachment injuries. The Four Quadrant Model and the Healthy Self-Actualizing Model can help identify the degree of effort the patient uses in an attempt to maintain psychic equilibrium. By breaking the psyche into four distinct quadrants, we can begin to see the systemic interconnection of the four quadrant sub-systems, as well as the degree to which patients split parts of each quadrant off from other parts. From an assessment standpoint, the more cut off the patient is from having an awareness of the relationship between aspects of each quadrant, the more intensely the patient will hold onto rigidly held beliefs, wishes, and assumptions.

A number of questions that you can use to determine the level of rigidity of the patient's defense structure are listed below.

- How amenable is the patient to receiving feedback?
- What is the quality and level of detail provided around self-disclosure?
- Which quadrants initially appear to be avoided or undeveloped, and which quadrants occupy most of the patient's concerns?
- How over-determined are the patient's efforts to succeed?
- Is there a compulsive quality to these efforts?
- What is the quality of the patient's personal self-care?
- What is the reaction when you bring the topic of self-care into the dialogue?
- What behaviors, feelings, areas of life seem to be minimized or avoided?
- How realistic are the patient's expectation of self and of others?
- What are the repeating patterns that seem to replay over and over again?
- What wishes and longings do you suspect underlie these repeated patterns?
- Where are there pockets of resilience, strength, and spontaneity?
- What are topic areas that seem to be off-limits or avoided?
- What is the patient's response to disappointment?
- How easily is it for the patient to forgive, to apologize, to learn from mistakes?
- What is the quality and extent of the patient's support system?

These questions are aimed at helping clinicians begin to formulate a working assessment of severity of pathology and areas of strength or resilience.

An accurate initial assessment helps set realistic treatment goals, increase understanding of the type of progress and the pace of you can expect to make, and it can help track outcomes of various intervention techniques.

If you examine the specific items listed within each quadrant of the Healthy Self Model, you can then compare this to the information gathered from an initial intake interview with a patient. Most of our patients fall somewhere on the continuum of health and illness. Many patients, however, are not aware of what specific qualities of healthy behavior might look like. By asking patients direct questions that pertain to items and qualities listed within the Healthy Self Model, the therapeutic dialogue can engage the patient's curiosity, opening discourse around new strategies for approaching problems, as well as uncovering wishes and longing that the patient has kept under the surface our outside of consciousness.

Identifying Repeating Patterns

The organizing schemas that comprise the foundation of character formation describe how one's sense of self comes into being. Defensively constructed organizing schemas are patterns of behavior that were early "solutions" or attempts at creating psychic stability. The lack of adequate relational attunement from the past often leaves a formidable residue of characterological damage that remains in the present due to varying degrees of trauma and/or deprivation. This residue of damage is *alive* to some degree in all of us and is revealed through the repetition of dysfunctional patterns that inhibit growth and require the expenditure of a great deal of psychic energy. The more consciously aware and the more curious we become about the underlying source that motivates these repeating patterns, the greater the likelihood that individuals can make different choices that lead to better outcomes.

Robert Stolorow (2013) describes defensively constructed organizing schemas as a consequence of traumatic 'malattunement between the child-caregiver interaffective system. He states,

> *One consequence of developmental trauma, relationally conceived, is that affect states take on enduring, crushing meanings. From recurring experiences of malattunement, the child acquires the unconscious conviction that unmet developmental yearnings and reactive painful feeling states are manifestations of a loathsome defect or of an inherent inner badness. A defensive self-ideal is often established, representing a self-image purified of the offending affect states that were perceived to be unwelcome or damaging to caregivers. Living up to this affectedly purified ideal becomes a central requirement for maintaining harmonious ties to others and for upholding self-esteem. Thereafter, the emergence of prohibited affect is experienced as a failure to embody the required ideal, an exposure of the underlying essential defectiveness or badness, and is accompanied by feelings of isolation, shame, and self-loathing, (p. 386)*

Stolorow's above description of developmental trauma as it applies to attachment injuries perfectly captures what has been highlighted, throughout this chapter, in our description of the Four Quadrant Model. Stolorow connects ruptures in attachment and consequent malattunement to the construction of a defensively based idealized self-structure, which is precisely at the heart of the Four Quadrant construct. The defensive ideal is in the service of protecting the self from essential defectiveness or badness in order that feelings of fear, isolation, and shame do not break through to the surface of consciousness.

This chapter began by introducing the question, "What are the qualities that comprise a healthy self?" Of course, health and the development of a healthy self must be viewed on a continuum. But how does one determine where the line gets crossed from relative health to what we would label as psychopathology? The emergence of symptoms is one indicator, but well before symptoms create enough psychic discomfort to prompt individuals to enter into therapy, we can spot compulsively driven behaviors and patterns that permeate the personality and interfere with the development of the authentic self. Ignoring these patterns, insisting that compulsively driven "solutions" will work, is what eventually lead to psychic distress.

Prior to the break-through of symptoms, the injured or *vulnerable aspects of the self* split into warring factions that are dissociated from each other and remain outside of conscious awareness. Without the protective mechanism of dissociative splitting, a fragmentation of self-integration would occur. Unfortunately, splitting also prevents the integration of parts of the self into the conscious narrative. While splitting serves a protective function of preventing psychic fragmentation, it does nothing to help resolve internalized conflicts. Self-defeating patterns will continue. The most damaging split occurs between the self-hating self that is divorced from the self-idealizing self that holds in contempt anything short of perfection. Thus, we see the compulsively driven push to prove self-worth. (Danielian & Gianotti, 2012, pp. 21–22.)

When conflicts remain unresolved, negative patterns or enactment will continue to repeat, often with little conscious recognition of the repetitive pattern. The two graphic models provided in this chapter enable clinicians to recognize splits more quickly between various parts of the personality. Specifically, the Four Quadrant Model helps clinicians recognize behaviors, beliefs, and expectations that are unrealistic, fantastical, or rigidly held. The model also enables clinicians to recognize patterns and approaches to life that continually result in exhaustion, disappointment, or the limitation of spontaneity, joy, and authenticity.

Engagement in therapy helps clients to eventually recognize reflexively repeating patterns. One of my clients involved in couples therapy refers to these repeating patterns as scripts or *"a thread that has always run through our relationship"*. After working in treatment for months, she was able to name the thread as mistrust. Having grown up with a mother who was hyper-critical and verbally abusive, she was always waiting for the other shoe to drop. As a child, she could be celebrating a success or enjoying an outing with her mother, when without provocation, her mother would turn on her and attack, destroying any good feeling between them. Thus, her fear, the thread that she brought into the present, was that her husband would react similarly. *"He's such a good salesman. I'm always convinced that he's using those skills to manipulate me, to get what he wants."* Although she could re-cognize that her assumptions about him were often unfair and unfounded, what was split off from consciousness was the affective memory of mistrust of her mother that was projected onto her husband. Once this connection between the split off part could be incorporated into her conscious awareness, her reflexive pattern of mistrust could be modified.

Three Dominant Trends in Organizing Schematics

One of the ways that the Four Quadrant Model can be applied clinically is to help us identify repeated defensively based patterns that manifest through present-day enactments. These relational enactments reveal an internalized organizing schematic of how individuals move through the world and their response to others. Therefore, the Four Quadrant Model not only reflects a picture of the beliefs, values, and over-determined efforts that individuals use to prove self-worth reflected in Quadrant One, the model also helps us capture repeated relational patterns that reveal how an individual's early attachment failures are carried into adulthood, as reflected in Quadrants Two, Three, and Four. These repeated relational patterns are somewhat predictable, and they contain elements that reflect:

• longings for redemption and release from pain and suffering,
• as well as an internalized guardedness and basic mistrust in others, created as a means of self-protection due to early attachment failures.

Both of the above dimensions of the individual's organizing schematic have a shared function – the avoidance of fully confronting and processing the reality of the grief and loss that resulted from the original attachment injury. The avoidance of grief (or affective collapse into psychic fragmentation) is what drives the over-compensation and over-idealized longing for rescue. It is also what recreates the dysfunctional pattern of mistrust, retaliation, and passive resignation. The unresolved tension within the psyche between longings for rescue in combination with the need for guardedness and self-protection is what constitutes the defense of psychic splitting. These splits manifest as repeated patterns or ways of moving through the world.

Karen Horney (1950) described these patterns as three dominant trends that become repeatedly enacted in relation to others. These trends or re-peating patterns largely fall outside of awareness. Depending upon the degree of attachment injury in childhood, these characterological patterns had the power to lead to greater and greater depletion of the self.

All of us possess all three trends but, under the weight of psychic conflict, one trend with its associated splits will typically become paramount, constantly driven by the unconscious attempt to achieve safety and prove self-worth. These human tendencies, when used as defensive over-compensations to keep feelings of shame or vulnerability split off, now fall into the pathological rather than normal realm. Elegant in their simplicity, Horney was able to capture these styles of relating to the world as: *moving toward people, moving against people, or moving away from people.*

Compulsively driven, these trends are inevitably accompanied by, and sustained by, unintegrated splits between self-contempt and unattainable perfection. These self-sustaining solutions perhaps implicate temperament but most certainly involve family environment, cultural conditioning, and psychic conflict. Needless to say, the degree and pervasiveness of the split determines the level of pathology and/or symptomatic thoughts, feelings, and behaviors (Danielian & Gianotti, 2012, pp. 29–30). A more detailed description of the three trends is described below.

Moving Toward People

The movement toward people is a pattern that Horney referred to as the *Compliant or Over-Attached Self-Effacing Solution.* Individuals with this style grew up in the cloud of someone else's shadow, most often a parent or sibling. Affection was attainable but only at a "price of self-subordinating devotion" (Horney, 1950, p. 222). Personal autonomy was thwarted in childhood, and self-credit became associated with something that was negative. Believing it presumptuous to even have an opinion, these individuals often will say, "I don't know" when asked a personal question about beliefs, dreams, or ambitions. Their life strategy is the belief that love will conquer all. Conscious assumptions or unconscious wishes work to undermine or denigrate one's own assets and accomplishments. Personal accomplishments, if they occur, are framed as luck or due to someone else's intervention. In the attempt to solve interpersonal conflict, these individuals seek security through the accomplishments of others, or through taking care of others.

The compulsivity behind this characterological pattern is that no amount of love, reassurance, or approval assuages the fear that the person is adequate enough, has done enough to be worthy of love. These individuals are continuously plagued by self-doubts, self-reproach, and self-denigration. However, they also are extremely sensitive to perceived slights and become wounded if they are overlooked or if praise for their efforts is not forthcoming. Retaliation around perceived slights often takes the form of tearful withdrawal, recrimination of self or others, or through cold, punishing silence.

Moving Against People

The Movement Against People is a pattern that Horney referred to as the *Expansive Solution: The Appeal of Mastery*. Individuals with this style primarily identify with the grandiose or glorified self. The appeal of life lies in mastering situations and bending them to their will, whether through the power of their intelligence, ambitious pursuits, or vindictive triumphs over others who are perceived to be adversaries. Such individuals openly covet self-sufficiency, ambition, aggressiveness, superiority, and triumph. Failures or rejection of their expansive efforts either lead to corrosive self-hate and self-contempt or attempts to regain the upper hand by devaluing, punishing, or bringing other people down. In childhood these individuals learned to believe that true affection was impossible to attain, therefore, self-worth was defined as becoming invulnerable to others and the self-righteous master of one's fate.

The compulsivity behind this characterological pattern lies in believing in the magic of greatness; therefore, all efforts are directed toward this aim. Disappointment is equated with defeat which threatens to uncover deeply buried feelings of shame and inadequacy. Acts of retaliation and revenge become a relied upon strategy to reestablish homeostatic balance as well as helping to distance from feelings of inadequacy, vulnerability, or the need to rely on others for help. It is also difficult for these individuals to receive any advice because the underlying belief is that they know more and are more intelligent than most people.

Moving Away from People

The Movement Away from People is a trend that Horney referred to as *Resignation: The Appeal of Freedom*. The compulsive drive in this third solution is to achieve a state of freedom and independence that is impervious to outside influence. In childhood and in adolescence, these individuals grew up in environments where they were coerced into obedience that was beyond tolerance. The solution to extreme parental coercion involved converting the self to an on-looker on life. Resignation from active involvement in living or in engagement with others creates a person who devalues attachment, a person who tries to avoid having any wishes or needs at all.

A profound aspect of such a personality is the exquisite sensitivity to being controlled or told what to do. This produces a sensitivity that often becomes so pervasive as to include moral indignation at someone invading his or her personal property, a fear of commitment, an avoidance of decision-making that would foreclose other options, and an intolerance for rules and regulations that confine personal liberties or threaten the fantasy of limitless possibilities. These individuals are thrown into endless internal debate, where moving in any direction might compromise integrity and individuality. Although they will comply with obvious rules, they quickly become the nay-sayers of any group that requires commitment or collective action.

The Impact on Treatment

Each of the above character solutions will have a direct impact on how the patient responds to treatment. Presenting problems and repeated patterns can be anticipated through the patient's predominant trend or defensive style, including:

• assumptions about therapy,
• issues of trust and mistrust,
• and the development of the therapeutic bond.

Resistance and enactments will initially or eventually play out based on the patient's predominant style. Understanding the motivating drivers of each style helps the therapist discern the types of questions to ask that will help guide the inquiry process and somewhat mitigate triggers of defensive guardedness or withdrawal. Although the therapeutic process inevitably will trigger old wounds and hidden places of shame and vulnerability, having an awareness of the patient's predominant pattern helps in the disruption and repair/restoration process. As Wolf (1988) explains, clients come to therapy with the hope that the therapist will be competent and fair-minded, but they also hold a fear around being misunderstood or unfairly judged. At some point in the therapeutic relationship, the therapist will inevitably disappoint or fail to meet the patient's expectations.

Once the patient experiences disappointment in the therapist and verbally expresses said disappointment, this is where the repair/restoration process can have an ameliorating effect on the client's character solution. It is at the point of therapeutic rupture that the therapist's task is to encourage discussion in an effort to understand, articulate, and repair disappointed expectations (Wolf, 1988, pp 110–111). It is out of this attempt to hear more about the patient's disappointed longings and expectations, coupled with the absence of defensive retaliation on the part of the therapist, that the patient can slowly begin to relinquish characterologically learned tendencies around self-protection and mistrust.

In terms of the three defensive solutions that Horney described, here is how each of these styles is likely to initially present within the unfolding therapeutic relationship:

For individuals with a style of *Moving Toward,* they are likely to initially present as a "the good patient", trying to please, being careful not to challenge the therapist or voice discomfort with the process. They will profusely apologize if they become ill or if an appointment has to be cancelled, or if they perceive that any accommodation to their needs might create an inconvenience. These patients enter therapy with expectations that the therapist will "fix" their problems or give recommendations that will magically relieve their symptoms, and they will *loyally wait* until the therapist provides the answer. Although they ask for suggestions or guidance, their follow-through on suggestions is often lacking or tentative.

Using the Four Quadrant Model as a reference point, individuals with the style of *Moving Toward* often have an under-developed sense of self. Therefore, spending time inquiring into dimensions that represent Quadrant One is worthy of attention. Also, since this style is overly caretaking of others, these patients often present with preoccupations around relational issues contained within Quadrant Three. Personal wishes and longings for attention are masked by worry about giving enough to others or sufficiently fulfilling their responsibilities to others. Issues that center around unfairness and lack of mutuality in relationship are initially minimized, and feelings of impatience or anger at being slighted are often denied. When the therapist directs inquiry about the patient's own needs, there is often confusion around legitimate needs vs. neediness. Personal needs are often framed as being selfish. Fear of rejection or abandonment is compensated for by making themselves invaluable to others. Quadrant Four largely remains under consciousness, and if displays of retaliation occur, they usually are in the form of turning against the self or silent withdrawal.

For individuals with the style of *Moving Against*, the need to prove competence and self-sufficiency remain paramount, even when they seek help from a therapist. Depending on the rigidity of the character style and the severity of the symptoms, individuals will present with varying degree of guardedness and/or suspicion around whether therapy will be of any value. Often an external trigger, whether that be interpersonal and/or workplace difficulties or a major disappointment or loss, will be the reason many of these patients enter treatment.

Patients' reactions to the therapist will often contain elements of over-valuing or devaluing. For example, a patient may be impressed with your credentials and feel that you measure up to their standards, allowing you into their circle of the chosen few, or the patient may make subtle comments that are devaluing or dismissive of the therapeutic process. The therapist may be criticized for not saying something "just right" or not grasping what the patient is trying to say. In either case, these patients experience feelings of vulnerability or being put in a position of needing help as shameful or weak. Therefore, the process of revealing painful material is often difficult for the therapist to access. These individuals often believe they are misunderstood, treated unfairly by others, or find other people's needs to be an annoyance or a sign of weakness.

Using the Four Quadrant Model as a reference guide, individuals with the style of *Moving Against* often present with an over-inflated sense of self-importance and entitlement. Quadrant One is highly developed in terms of confidence of one's convictions, however, the beliefs, values, and motivations that drive over-determined efforts to succeed typically remain under-examined. Self-righteousness takes the place of self-reflection and humility. Therefore, asking questions that lead to increasing the patient's curiosity and tolerating differences of opinion are helpful. When working on the relational level in Quadrant Three, a discernment process is needed to determine whether patients have over-inflated expectations of an idealized other who will meet their every need, heal old wounds, and by-pass a grieving process, or the therapist must determine whether the patient lacks empathy, desiring to meet his/her own needs at the expense of the other. In either pattern there is a lack of realistic expectations and an inability to achieve mutuality within relationships. Therefore, leading the dialogic exchange toward focusing on issues of fairness or uncovering unrequited longings that are split off from conscious awareness can help break the cycle of repeated disappointments in relationship. Disappointed expectations lead to retaliation, including negative transferential responses, that can range from subtle devaluing statements to outbursts of rage, to bolting from treatment. Therefore, recognizing and palpating negative transferential communications that stem from Quadrant Four as they begin to surface, rather than ignoring subtle comments, can help prevent more extreme forms of negative transference from boiling up in the future.

Individuals who enter therapy with the style of *Moving Away* will often be verbally forthcoming and will not hold back from expressing an opinion or stating what is on their mind. They will also be respectful of the boundaries of therapy, such as being on time and abiding by cancellation policies. However, the therapeutic relationship seems to create little impact emotional resonance during sessions. In addition, the content of material that is discussed doesn't seem to be assimilated or remembered from session to session. Often, therapists can feel invisible or unimportant, because for these patients, reliance on others is frightening as it threatens to confine their sense of unlimited freedom. Therefore, one theme that provides an opening for therapeutic exploration is the powerful appeal of freedom. Freedom and independence are highly prized and create an internalized sense of security that is symbolized both psychologically and philosophically. Entering into a conversation focusing on Quadrant One, where the therapist shows a genuine interest in trying to understand the importance of remaining independent and self-reliant, allows for a relaxing of hypervigilance around the fear that he/she will be analyzed or reduced to a diagnosis containing negative judgment.

One way to access the inner life of these patients is often through the interpretation of their dreams that are often filled with conflicts, fears, and passions that remain under the surface. Using the Four Quadrant Model to help understand and interpret conflicts and fears can be a useful road map. In childhood individuals with the style of *Moving Away* were often coerced by parental forces, where extremes of attention coupled with abuse sent mixed messages about trust and the reliability of attachment figures. In some cases, these individuals may have suffered from a reversal of the parent-child relationship, where caretaking of the adult was coupled with messages of guilt if the child did not comply. Given these possible attachment patterns, focusing on Quadrant Three and Quadrant Four would be useful. For example, encouraging patients to talk about the rules of engagement with early attachment figures (Q3) and giving permission to voice feelings of anger or unfairness (Q4) is a way that the treatment process can be constructively engaged.

Summary

In summary, the Four Quadrant Model and the three characterological trends that Karen Horney described can give the therapist an expanded understanding of "sub-system splits". The Four Quadrant Model helps to illustrate how the interpersonal and intrapsychic aspects of the self are interconnected and how feelings of shame are the driving force behind repeated patterns. Because all defensive postures or solutions are compulsively driven and remain largely out of awareness, the major objective of using the model is to illustrate how sub-systems splits interact and reinforce a homeostatic, systemic balance. The Four Quadrant Model in comparison with the Healthy Self-Actualizing Model can reveal where the therapeutic dialogue can create leverage to penetrate unconscious or under-developed thoughts, feelings, and longings contained within and between the quadrants. Pointing out features of healthy self-actualization can have an impact on dismantling defensive response patterns in the service of integration and healing.

The utility of these two models is that they can serve as a template to help track the intersubjective exchange between the therapist and the patient in any given moment. Therefore, using these models as a way of staying in the intersubjective present, grounds theory more firmly in the phenomenology of experience. This then can be seen as a natural unfolding of relational process dynamics in the service of historical and personal integration (Danielian & Gianotti, 2012, p. 32). Karen Horney (1950) described alienation from the 'true self' as the origin of most psychic distress and described the true self as "the 'original' force toward individual growth and fulfillment" (p. 158). In a state of natural functioning, adaptive skills and resilience emerge. According to Horney (1950), this true self is an "intrinsic potentiality" or "central inner force, common to all human beings" (p. 17) one that is the core source of development. Similarly, Donald Winnicott believed that much of psychopathology is a "result of an inflation of the false self and a corresponding under-development of a true self" (Ryan & Deci, 2017, p. 59).

References

Adler, A. (1930). *The science of living*. Allen & Unwin.

Allport, G. W. (1943). The ego in contemporary psychology. *Psychology Review, 50*(5), 451–478.

Allport, G. W. (1950). *The nature of personality: Selected papers*. Addison Wesley.

Bellak, L., & Sheehy, M. (1976). The broad role of ego function and assessment. *American Journal of Psychiatry, 133*(11), 1259–1264.

Bion, W. R. (1962). *Learning from experience*. Heinnemann.

Bion, W. R. (1963). *Elements of psycho-analysis*. Heinnemann.

Danielian, J., & Gianotti, P. (2012). *Listening with purpose: Entry points into shame and narcissistic vulnerability*. Routledge

Erickson, E. H. (1950). *Childhood and society*. W. W. Norton.

Fairbairn, W. R. D. (1952). *Psychoanalytic studies of the personality*. Tavistock Publications.

Fredrickson, B. L., & Losada, M. F. (2005). Positive affect and the complex dynamics of human flourishing. *American Psychologist, 60*(7), 678–686.

Freud, S. (1905). Three essays on the theory of sexuality. *American Journal of Psychiatry, 148* (12), 1733–1735.

Freud, S. (1926). *Inhibition, symptoms, and anxiety*. W. W. Norton & Company, Inc.

Gfellner, B. M., & Cordoba, A. I. (2017). Identity problems, ego strengths, perceived stress, and adjustment during contextual changes at university. *Identity: An International Journal of Theory and Research, 17*(1), 25–39.

Gianotti, P., & Danielian, J. (2017). *Uncovering the resilient core: A workbook on the treatment of narcissistic defenses, shame, and emerging authenticity*. Routledge.

Goldberg, A., & Stepansky P. E. (Eds.) (1984). *How does analysis cure?* University of Chicago Press.

Guntrip, H. (1971). *Psychoanalytic theory, therapy, and the self*. Basic Books.

Hartmann, H. (1958). Ego psychology and the problem of adaptation. *Journal of the American Psychoanalytic Association Monograph Series: Vol. 1.* (D. Rapaport, Trans.). International Universities Press, Inc.

Hartmann, H., Kris, E., & Loewenstein R. M. (1964). Papers on psychoanalytic psychology. *Psychological Issues Monograph, 4*(2).

Hayes, S. C., Wilson, K. G., Gifford, E. V., Follette, V. M., & Strosahl, K. (1996). Experiential avoidance and behavioral disorders: A functional dimensional approach to diagnosis and treatment. *Journal of Consulting and Clinical Psychology, 64*(6), 1152–1168.

Horney, K. (1950). *Neurosis and human growth: The struggle toward self-realization*. Norton.

Kagle, A., & Levay, A. N. (1977). Ego deficiencies in the areas of pleasure, intimacy, and cooperation: Guidelines in the diagnosis and treatment of sexual dysfunctions. *Journal of Sex & Marital Therapy, 3*(1), 10–18.

Kashdan, T. B., & Rottenberg, J. (2010). Psychological flexibility as a fundamental aspect of health. *Clinical Psychology Review, 30*(11), 865–878.

Klein, M. (1952). Some theoretical conclusions regarding the emotional life of the infant. In *Envy and gratitude and other works 1946–1963* (pp. 61–93). The Free Press.

Klein, M., & Riviere, J. (1964). *Love, hate and reparation*. Norton.

Kohut, H. (1971). *The analysis of the self: A systematic approach to the psychoanalytic treatment of narcissistic personality disorders*. International Universities Press.

Kohut, H. (1977). *The restoration of the self*. International Universities Press.

Mahler, M. S., Pine, F., & Bergman, A. (1975). *The psychological birth of the human infant: Symbiosis and individuation.* Hutchinson & Co.

Markstrom, C., & Marshall, S. (2006). The psychosocial inventory of ego strengths: Examination of theory and psychometric properties. *Journal of Adolescence, 30*(1), 63–79.

Metz. J. R. (1961). A method for measuring aspects of ego strength. *Journal of Projective Techniques, 25*(4), 457–470.

Mitchell, S. A. (1993). *Hope and dread in psychoanalysis.* Harper Collins.

Mitchell, S. A., & Black, M. J. (1995). *Freud and beyond: A history of modern psycho analytic thought.* Basic Books.

Mitchell, S. A. (1997). *Influence and autonomy in psychoanalysis.* Analytic Press.

Ornstein, P. (Ed). (1978). *The search for the self: Selected writings of Heinz Kohut 1950–1978,* Vol. 1. International Universities Press.

Peterson, C., & Seligman, M. E. P. (2004). *Character strengths and virtues: A handbook of classification.* Oxford University Press.

Rapaport, D. (1950). On the psycho-analytic theory of thinking. *International Journal of Psychoanalysis, 31,* 161–170.

Ryan, R. M., & Deci, E. L. (2017). *Self-determination theory: Basic psychological needs in motivation.* The Guilford Press.

Seligman, M. E. (2004). *Character strengths and virtues: A Handbook and classification, Vol. 2.* Oxford University Press.

Stolorow, R. D. (2013). Intersubjective-systems theory: A phenomenological-contextualist psychoanalytic perspective. *Psychoanalytic Dialogues, 23,* 383–389. Routledge: Taylor & Francis Group.

Vallerand, R. J., Blanchard, C. M., Mageau, G. A., Koestner, R., Ratelle, C., Léonard, M., Gagné, M., & Marsolais, J. (2003). Les passions de l'âme: On obsessive and harmonious passion. *Journal of Personality and Social Psychology. 85*(4), 756–767.

Wachtel, P. (2008). *Relational theory and the practice of psychotherapy.* The Guilford Press.

Winnicott, D. W. (1951). Transitional objects and transitional phenomena. In *Through paediatrics to psychoanalysis* (pp. 229–242). Basic Books.

Winnicott, D. W. (1958). The capacity to be alone. In *The maturational processes and the facilitating environment* (pp. 29–36). International Universities Press.

Winnicott, D. W. (1960a). The theory of the parent-infant relationship. In *The maturational processes and the facilitating environment* (pp. 37–55). International Universities Press.

Winnicott, D. W. (1960b). Ego distortion in terms of true and false self. In *The maturational processes and the facilitating environment* (pp. 140–152). International Universities Press.

Wolf, E. S. (1988). *Treating the self: Elements of clinical self psychology.* The Guilford Press.

2 Understanding the Power of Loyalty Contracts: How to Recognize, Articulate, and Interrupt Repeated Patterns of Early Relational Failures

Introduction

Let us go back in time to set the scene – we are in one of the grand parlors of Buckingham Palace, on the eve of the Royal Wedding of Charles and Diana. It is dark in the elegantly appointed room, and fireworks are going off outside the palace in anticipation of the celebration to come. Charles is standing in the dark, staring out the window, uncertain whether to go forward with the wedding because he is in love with another.

(Enter Queen Elizabeth, who interrupts the silence)

When your Great Grandmother, Queen Mary, was a beautiful young princess, she was about to marry her Prince Charming, but before they got to the church he fell ill and died. But everyone had been so impressed with her that they put her together with his younger brother. Only one problem, the younger brother was Prince Charm-less… dull and shy. There was no attraction, certainly no love. But in order to make the marriage work, they were encouraged to focus on the bigger idea – DUTY. They worked, and worked, and worked. And out of that work a tiny seed grew, a seed of respect and admiration, a seed that grew into a flower they could eventually call love. They were married for 42 years. They stabilized the country that was at war with itself, and they left the crown stronger, while all around them great monarchies fell.

Now I cannot claim to be the most intuitive mother, but I do think I know when one of my children is unhappy. Whatever wretchedness you are feeling now, whatever doubts you harbor, if you could follow the example of your Great Grandmother, love and happiness will surely follow (The Crown, Season 4: Episode 3; Morgan et al., 2020)

Every family comes with its expectations, perhaps not on public display quite as much as the royal family. However, familial as well as cultural expectations are the cornerstone of what shapes our identity, becoming a powerful force that runs through the veins of us all. This chapter will focus on the themes of duty and loyalty, specifically as they connect to our

DOI: 10.4324/9781003120278-3

understanding of the relationship between Quadrant One and Quadrant Three. Recognizing the factors that reinforce the interconnection between these two quadrants is what allows us to better understand what compels our patients to make life decisions that are primarily reflexive, driven by familial and systemic forces that continue to be reinforced throughout the life span. These acknowledged and unacknowledged forces function as an over-arching organizing schema, one that takes the form of Learned Loyalty Contracts.

Loyalty Contracts can be conceptualized as an internalized system of beliefs, feelings, reactions, and expectations that were created and deeply rooted in early parent-child interactions as well as the particular experience of a person's socio-cultural context. Loyalty Contracts reflect the spoken or unspoken rules that one must obey in order to remain safe, preserve relational connection, and develop a sense of personal value. From an early age, children internalize those beliefs and expectations. For example, in the case of gender socialization – before the child is even born, we ask if the child is a boy or girl, and the minute we hear the answer, it's as if we set in motion a series of expectations and assumptions that both limit and shape the child's identity.

Relational patterns that develop and play out through the defensively based construction of the Four Quadrant Model affect the individual's sense of self (Q1) as well as their expectations, fears, and longings with regard to relational connection (Q3). Understanding the connection and interaction between these two quadrants in terms of the development of self and self-in-relationship provides the therapist with a better grasp of potential enactments, enactments that may occur within the therapeutic relationship as well as the patient's interactions in the outside world.

When family rules, messages, and expectations are fair, loving, consistent, and applied equally to all members, children will likely grow up with a sense of confidence in their own abilities, a trust in others, a general sense of optimism, and the capacity for mutuality in adult relationships. Unhealthy loyalty contracts, on the other hand, are comprised of rules and expectations that were often unfair, harsh, abusive, depriving, or inconsistent. The result is that these children will form varying degrees of insecure and/or disorganized attachment patterns.

Depending on the degree of trauma and/or deprivation in the family and the culture at large, most children who grow up in family environments with unhealthy loyalty contracts carry secret, internalized longings for rescue. At the same time, the reverse is also true. There is a fear of breaking free of the old loyalty contract, based on a belief that the child isn't worthy of something better, or s/he believes that no one can really be trusted. What is noteworthy is that the child's confusion and fear that are the result of early attachment failures go underground – encoded as unformulated experiences that later manifest through enactments in the therapist/client relationship.

In 1949 Ferenczi cogently described the internal state of children who were unable to establish a secure attachment, and he referred to this as a *Confusion of Tongues Between Adults and the Child*. Ferenczi writes, "These children feel physically and morally helpless, their personalities are not sufficiently consolidated in order to be able to protest, even if only in thought, for the overpowering force and authority of the adult makes them dumb and can rob them of their senses. *The same anxiety, however, if it reaches a certain maximum, compels them to subordinate themselves like automata to the will of the aggressor...* When the child recovers from such an attack, he feels enormously confused, in fact, split - and his confidence in the testimony of his own senses is broken (p. 162 italics in original.)

In other words, an unhealthy loyalty contract is the enacted embodiment of a *Confusion of Tongues,* one that represents the suffering, the struggles, and the longings contained within a child's brokenness. Yet, these feeling states cannot be accurately understood or integrated into the personality because they remain unformulated or split off. Donnel Stern (1997) reminds us that our patients begin to see, understand, and integrate split off parts of the self by first having a "benign other" reflect to them our own experience of being with them. This is the kind of therapeutic mirroring that Kohut (1977) refers to as − acknowledging aspects of the self that are necessary in order for our clients to be able to claim parts of themselves that had been unacknowledged or forbidden to exist. Understanding the value of working with loyalty contracts is what enables the therapist to integrate unformulated experiences into the personality, thus freeing up and claiming part of the self that had been unacknowledged or forbidden to exist.

Loyalty Contracts, Shame, and the Four Quadrant Model

Loyalty contracts can be recognized in the present moment by observing and tracking our clients' compulsively driven patterns and beliefs. By listening to the quality and/or rigidity of our clients' goals, their wishes, longings, and expectations in relationship, coupled with how they respond to repeated experiences of disappointment, we are able to see how childhood loyalty contracts shaped the personality. For example, we may observe a client's tentativeness, impulsivity, anger or ambivalence and wonder what parental rules helped shape these responses. Repeated patterns of behavior in adulthood reflect the core struggle contained within the unfair loyalty contract, regardless of whether the child (now adult) consciously desires to please the parent by remaining loyal and obedient to the contract. In a sense this struggle represents a psychic split, where the individual is at a loss as to how to maintain connection with a parent while at the same time moving forward toward authentically integrated self-expression. This pattern is also a dilemma in the greater cultural context. Most people of color in this society have been fed the steady messages about their inferiority on multiple levels. They too are a loss at how to be in relationship with a powerful other while trying to move forward toward thriving or authentic self-expression.

Loyalty contracts also represent a conflict or tension between wishes and longings for rescue coupled with an unconscious prohibition about breaking free due to complicated feelings of attachment guilt if the person leaves the "broken parent" behind. These feelings of guilt are often linked with a deeply held belief that no one can be really trusted, so why bother even daring to believe that finding a better relationship, creating a better life is possible. Yet, regardless of deeply embedded hopelessness, hidden longings for rescue remain. That is because most individuals who grew up with insecure attachments know at some core level that something wasn't right.

More often than not, blame for what wasn't right in childhood is turned inward. When children blame themselves for attachment/cultural failures, they will work harder to please, to fix a situation while, simultaneously, feeling a sense of shame or unworthiness. Here is where over-determined efforts become manifest in Quadrant One. As adults, these individuals have a continued need to prove self-worth because their childhood feelings of inadequacy remain. On the interpersonal level all children are wired to connect; but for children with insecure attachments, they find no clear pathway of how to do so (Quadrant Three). Therefore, these adults carry forward the longing for connection which can take the form of wishing for rescue by an over-idealized attachment figure – whether that be an intimate partner, teacher, mentor, political figure, or clergyperson. Alternately, the wish for comfort and reassurance can also take the form of latching onto rigid ideologies, where absolute answers or purity of sacrifice can serve as a stabilizing function within the personality. The search for answers and validation outside the self provides a psychic function of preserving hope – the hope that finding the perfect other will erase the individual's internal turmoil of past pain and uncertainty.

What is noteworthy is that in most cases loyalty contracts are either poorly known or they are accepted as normal, where the patient adopts an attitude of "this is just the way things are." Isabel Wilkerson explains, "Perhaps it is the unthinking acquiescence, the blindness to one's imprisonment, that is the most effective way for human being to remain captive. People who do not know they are captive will not resist their bondage, (2020, p. 34)." Despite the frequent repetition of dysfunctional patterns coupled with repeated disappointment, most individuals with varying degrees of attachment disorders seem to have an absence of curiosity as to why these disappointments continue to occur.

In childhood, parental dictates that shaped and monitored the unfair loyalty contract prohibited discussion or negotiation between the parent and child. Therefore, as these individuals mature into adulthood, they often have under-developed self-reflective capacities. Without curiosity and the capacity for self-reflection, they are unable to question, interrupt, or modify their dysfunctional patterns. The irony here is loyalty contracts are one of the most significant driving forces in a person's life, and yet they are probably one of the most underexamined aspects of human interaction.

The underbelly that drives the repeated continuation of an old loyalty contract is the client's internalized beliefs and fears which are operating as conscious and unconscious drivers in Quadrant One and Quadrant Three. For example, a client may be hesitant to pursue self-interests or ambitions in Quadrant One because of harbored fears that the partner will become angry and/or threaten to leave the relationship. In this case, individual needs in Quadrant One become secondary to the need for connection and security in Quadrant Three. Or a client's belief about self in Quadrant One (I'm not really worthy of something better) will often determine what a client will settle for in relationships in Quadrant Three.

A poignant example of this is a young black girl who is raised by an inconsistently attuned mother and a father who is very limited and often frightens her with his chronic rage-filled dysregulation. She hears from an early age how dark she is and how much she does not look like her mother. Seeing lighter skinned or white children who are considered prettier and better, she internalizes a sense of ugliness and unworthiness. Fast forward into adulthood, she is only attracted to light-skinned or white men, and she gives to them and cares for them regardless of how they treat her. Longing for rescue, she believes that somehow these relationships will redeem her because she believes that she will never be able to find someone who is caring and kind to love her. Thus, the internalized messages of the early loyalty contract repeat without full examination, understanding, resolution, or liberation from the shame.

What all loyalty contracts have in common is that regardless of the degree of unfairness of the contract, the spoken and unspoken rules and expectations contained within the relationship between the parent and child have been deeply embedded and reinforced over years of interaction. Abiding by the rules are directly connected to the child's sense of value and membership in the family unit and the culture at large. This is especially true in situations where clients have been assigned the role of protecting the parent, where the "goodness" of the child was defined by remaining in a protective role. The challenge of dismantling this form of the loyalty contract can be more difficult. This is often because the act of separation results in further dysfunction or decline on the part of the parent, thus, reinforcing the client's sense of disloyalty and betrayal.

Loyalty Contracts as a "Quid Pro Quo" Engagement

A further way to understand the power of loyalty contracts is to think about them as quid pro quo arrangements. For example, a mother's verbal and non-verbal messages might convey this – "If you keep your needs to yourself, become completely self-sufficient, and not ask me for anything, then I'll tell you that you are a brilliant and wonderful child because you will make me feel proud, and I won't feel so anxious and overwhelmed by life. But, if you challenge me or whine and complain, I will tell you that you are inconsiderate and selfish, that you only care about yourself and you don't care about me. And that will be your fault because look how you've upset me. Now, I feel horrible about myself and horrible about you. I'll retreat into tears, or I will give you the cold shoulder, and I will threaten to withdraw my love if you don't straighten up and behave as I say you must."

Obviously, a young, vulnerable child will do anything to try to maintain love and connection. Imagine the fear, confusion, and shame associated with early verbal and non-verbal parental cues that are based on a child's acceptance only being measured by how well that child attends to the parents' needs. Children cannot afford to question the parameters of the loyalty contract because to do so would be dangerous and emotionally dysregulating. Therefore, parental messages become accepted as the truth, reflected in beliefs about *who I am* and about *how I must behave* in relationship. Because these messages are internalized at such an early and vulnerable stage of development, they often remain unquestioned in adulthood and play out through similar enactments later in life. In this way, loyalty contracts become a predominant factor in the organizing schematics of the psyche.

In most unfair loyalty contracts if the contract is broken, the parent feels justified to punish the child by pulling away and withdrawing love, or through verbal or physical abuse. Parental retaliation remains unquestioned, justifiable in the mind of adults because the parents' narcissistic investment in maintaining the rules also remains largely outside of their own conscious awareness. The invisible or unspoken power of unfair loyalty contracts lies in child's vulnerability and need to maintain connection. There is no allowance for the child to challenge whether the rules are unhealthy, unfair, or impossible to achieve. The contract may be confusing for the child; it may feel painful, and frightening, but it is accepted as a given because it is all that the child knows. For example, if a parent has an over-driven standard of perfectionism, the falseness of perfectionism never gets questioned. The child will either attempt to over-achieve to meet this standard, or s/he will feel shamed and inadequate when missing the mark. Either outcome interferes with authentic self-emergence.

The grid in Figure 2.1 illustrates the quid pro quo formula of most unfair loyalty contracts. Obviously, there are degrees of rigidity and punitive retaliation in the spoken and unspoken rules of engagement.

This grid is provided to help understand the various components that shape the formation of unfair loyalty contracts, particularly highlighting how parts of the authentic self must be sacrificed to preserve a sense of safety and belonging. However, understanding the powerful grip of the

---

If I keep this contract

1. If I do ____(A)____, then this ____(B)____ will happen (expected outcome), and it will mean (learned assigned meaning): this about Me ____(C)____ and this will mean ____(D)____about our relationship (interpretation of self and relationship).

> 1. *(A) If I'm real quiet and make myself invisible when daddy comes home, (B) then he won't hit me or yell at mommy; (C) this will mean that I'm a good boy, (D) and this will make everybody safe and happy.*

If I break this contract

2. If I do anything other than ____(A)____, (if I break the loyalty contract) then this ____(X)____ will happen (expected outcome), and it will mean (learned assigned meaning) this ____(Y)____ about Me and this about Us ____(Z)____ (interpretation of self and relationship).

> 2. *(A) If I do anything other than be quiet and invisible, (X) then daddy will start yelling and blaming me or mommy, (Y) then this will mean that it's my fault that mommy is crying, and (Z) why I deserve to be punished and go to bed without supper.*

Figure 2.1 Quid Pro Quo Formula.

patient's sacrifice runs the risk of becoming lost if you try to apply this illustration in a concrete, formulaic way. It is better to remain attuned to the patient's internalized assumptions and their repeated, over-determined patterns to help formulate their loyalty contract.

Asking the patient specific questions about the rules of their family of origin may help you discover the patient's internalized assumptions as well as conflicts they may have between self-advocacy and relational connection. Asking questions is also a way to guard against using the quid-pro-quo formula from becoming reified or too concrete.

Crafting the Loyalty Contract Using the Therapist's Counter-Transferential Experience

Another way you can imagine what it might have been like for patients growing up is to reflect upon what it feels like to be in the room with them. You can gain access to parental expectations by getting a clearer sense of what the patient expects of you by asking yourself:

- *What does it feel like sitting in the room with this patient?*
- *Do you feel any pressure to "do something" for the patient?*

- *Is this a demand that the patient expresses directly, or is it a feeling you're picking up on?*
- *What are you afraid will happen if you disappoint this patient?*

In adulthood, patients will initially or eventually replicate their learned loyalty contract with the therapist. This can happen in a number of ways. Patients may simply repeat the same learned behavior and remain "dutiful" to the original loyalty contract, projecting onto the therapist the same fears and judgments that the parents demonstrated. Or patients may do the complete opposite and assume a demanding/aggressive parental role and place these expectations onto the therapist as a means of finally getting their needs met.

Let us say you have a client who has been through a number of therapists. She is an overachiever at work, suffers from anxiety, is highly intellectualized, and floods the therapy session with continual talk. She is quick to lash out at others that she deems to be inferior but will quickly turn her disappointment against herself if she perceives that others are better than she is.She has read numerous self-help books and wants to find the answer to achieve happiness in her relationships with her female friends. It is difficult for the therapist to interject any comments, and the therapist is beginning to feel frustrated and drained by the therapy.

In one of our consultation groups, we crafted the patient's loyalty contract demands that were aimed at the therapist. Here are two examples. The first is more straightforward, and the second highlights the quadrants that are at play within the loyalty contract demand.

> *It's your job to listen to me and tell me all the answer so I won't have to feel anxious, and if you don't, I get to leave you and it means you're incompetent – it's your fault not mine.*

> *These are the skills I need – (overcompensation – Q1 insistence). You need to give me the skills so I can have perfect relationships (wish not grounded in reality – Q3). Having perfect relationships would mean I would never be disappointed. However, if you do disappointment me and don't give me what I'm asking for, you're just like all the rest of them (devaluing – Q4), and I'm going to leave you before you can leave me.*

Once the loyalty contract was articulated from the therapist's countertransferential feeling state, the patient's original loyalty contract with her parents came into clearer view. Our consultation group was able to image what it must have been like to grow up in her family; they were able to feel the constriction and the harsh demands that were placed on the patient once the loyalty contract had been translated into words. The therapist was then able to get in touch with the patient's very real cry that had remained unspoken – the hope that someone would finally make her feel cared for her in the way that she deserved, that someone would teach her how to negotiate the world so that she would feel less alone. This exercise re-activated the therapist's compassion, enabling her to speak to the feelings and needs that were under the surface.

Clearly, how therapists respond to their own counter-transferential cues is an ongoing exchange that is dependent upon and shaped by the patient and therapist's intersubjective vulnerabilities. Patient's overt or covert expectations often trigger areas of therapists' vulnerabilities, vulnerabilities that are stimulated by their own learned loyalty contracts. For example, if the therapist has to take a break from sessions due to complications from an unexpected surgery, the client might state, *"I'm feeling abandoned by you. I know that doesn't sound fair. But now I'm worried about you, and I'm angry that I have to worry because now that means I have to take care of you, and I don't like it."* If the therapist happens to be feeling guilty about taking so much time off or if his/her own loyalty contract meant you could never disappoint your parents, the therapist may say, *"Well, it's not like I had any choice in the matter,"* rather than staying with the client's honest reflections of being thrown into an old dilemma of being disappointed with an early parental figure. (Note: Further elaboration on how loyalty contracts play out within the intersubjective landscape of therapist-patient interaction will be covered in Chapter Seven on Transference.)

Understanding Loyalty Contracts as a Conflict Between Dependence and Independence

An important question for therapists to ask themselves is what are the factors that determine whether a parent/child relationship will lead to the consolidation of a healthy sense of self vs. a disrupted sense of self coherence? In families where there is a scarcity of psychic resources, if there isn't enough emotional bandwidth to go around leading to chaos and instability, the fundamental parent/child dyad can deteriorate into a competition for whose needs will be met. With a fragile or exhausted parent, the question is whether the infant's needs will overwhelm/devour the parent, or whether the parent's need for self-preservation will lead to neglecting the baby in order to preserve his/her own sense of self-coherence or need satisfaction.

Jessica Benjamin (1988) in her studies on domination and submission, states that the conflict between dependence and independence, power and surrender can be traced to the parent-infant relationship. In dysfunctional attachment configurations, the parent-child interaction does not allow for the necessary tension between self-assertion and mutual recognition, a delicate balance that is necessary for the self and other to meet as sovereign equals. She concludes that the development of a healthy sense of self stems from the need for recognition. We come to know who we are by being "the doer" in the shared company of another person who recognizes our actions, feelings, intentions, existence, and independence. When a parent is incapable of allowing for mutuality, a negative cycle of recognition is created, where the only way to assert one's autonomy is by obliterating the intrusive other, and the only way to achieve attunement and connection is by surrendering to the other (p. 28). In other words, the quid pro quo of extreme negative cycles of recognition, or the most primitive of unhealthy loyalty contracts, means that only one can be given to, only one can exist. Mutuality is not remotely possible.

Infant researchers (Beebe, et al, 2010; Beebe & Lachmann, 1988; Lyons-Ruth, 1999; Stern, 1985, 1989; Tronick, 1989) confirm Benjamin's clinical observations. In dysfunctional attachment patterns, rather than the following a "serve and return" pattern where parents take cues from the infant and reciprocate with recognition and delight, a pattern of "chase and dodge" may ensue in unhealthy response patterns. In these instances, the parent becomes the looming, coercive adult, and the child must either push away or surrender. In situations where attunement is ruptured, the delicate balance of mutual recognition is shattered.

Benjamin (2018) refers to various degrees of the pattern of "chase and dodge" as a primary experience of "doer and done to." In these instances, the parent is generally in the position of the "doer" and the child in a defensive posture of "done to." Depending on the severity of and frequency of misattunement, of "chase and dodge" without the attendant moments of repair, the child learns to sacrifice self-assertion through capitulation or dissociative shut-down. Although Tronick (1989) reminds us that all parent/child relationships have moments of rupture, the importance of repair is critical to restabilize the arousal state of the child, shifting away from hyper (obliteration) or hypo (surrendered) arousal states. Tronick (2007) has observed that when babies begin to move away from a parent, this may be a signal that they are in a state of over-stimulation or rupture. Healthy cuing responses from the parent must include recognizing potential ruptures and working toward repair. Tronick and Gold (2020) state that developing states of mutual attunement involves a series of rupture and repair, or disruption and repair.

As therapists when we develop further understanding of the nuanced components of intersubjective reality, we realize that we must adopt a stance of continuous accommodation in order to attend to possible ruptures in the therapeutic bond. Catching possible ruptures enables the work of therapeutic repair of the relational connection. This back-and-forth process dynamic of rupture and repair is what allows the relationship to develop more resilience, as the client experiences consistency and continuity in the face of disappointment/relational fractures.

Benjamin (2018) speaks of this clinical position as "the Third," and she defines this as the therapist's ability to hold and recognize the client as a "like subject." In other words, the idea of a neutral or "expert" position on the part of the therapist is called into question. The position of the Third is created through adopting a stance of deep and abiding respect for the patient, which creates a holding environment where the therapist can acknowledge the tension between both difference and sameness, where both parties' feelings and intentions can be shared. If there is a disruption in this delicate balance, relational repair requires that the caregiver [therapist] acknowledge–in deeds and communicative gestures—the violations of expected patterns of soothing or responsiveness, (p. 6). This unfolding dynamic process may not always feel smooth or harmonious, but repair is a critical component of surviving inevitable breakdowns in recognition. In the clinical situation the repair of dysfunctional loyalty contracts involves recognizing and understanding how early rules of engagement may trigger our client's distress. Tronick (1989) states that this recognition of infant distress is the most predictive factor in creating a secure attachment.

Privilege and Marginalization as a Social Construction of a Loyalty Contract

If we were to broaden the scope of understanding the impact that loyalty contracts have on us both individually and collectively, it is important to view these spoken and unspoken rules through the lens of "the contextual self" (Wachtel, 2014). From a larger systemic vantage point, loyalty contracts represent the collectively agreed upon rules of societal engagement, rules that enforce a particular system of loyalty that is shaped by and in the service of maintaining the status quo of power and privilege. Domination is at the heart of all unfair loyalty contracts. The "doer," whether that be the parent, the boss, the wealthy educated person of privilege, is allowed to play by rules that are in the service of maintaining power and control; they are not in the service of mutuality and support. The "done to" are meant to obey, whether that be the child, the student, the elderly, the intellectually challenged, the person of color, of poverty, or any identity we consider separate from those who hold power.

People in positions of subordination are not to question the status quo, which means they are to assume a subordinate position indefinitely. Just as unhealthy family loyalty contracts reflect the micro-enactment of power and domination, the social construction of collective unhealthy loyalty contracts reflect the expression of power and domination on a macro-level. One reinforces the other. And thus, the internalization of privilege and marginalization continues in an unbroken cycle – where shame denied and shame internalized on both sides of the equation – wield an unconscious, habituated grip on the soul.

Isabel Wilkerson (2020) refers to this collective social construction, this habituated grip, as a caste system. Caste systems, much like unfair loyalty contracts, are hierarchical in nature. They are not necessarily intentionally or consciously unfair. They are simply accepted as normal. Wilkerson states, "Caste is insidious and therefore powerful because it is not hatred, it is not necessarily personal. It is the worn grooves of comforting routines and unthinking expectations, patterns of a social order that have been in place for so long that it looks like the natural order of things" (p. 70). Those in the dominant group of any caste (or loyalty system) have an investment in keeping the hierarchy in place because when you position yourself above others, you maintain the benefits of respect, status, and privilege. White privilege, on the other hand, is based on the mere fact that being white promises the hope of eventual entre into a privileged position regardless of socioeconomic status.

Janet Helms (2020) states that, "Being accepted as White requires White people to acculturate to White culture where acculturate means to learn the rules, customs, and principles of Whiteness. If one acculturates or appears to do so in public, then one is accepted in many White environments" (p. 16). Members of disenfranchised or minoritized groups can never be acculturated into customs and principles of Whiteness because color doesn't disappear, in spite of one's material, political, or intellectual success. Survival and sense of identity, therefore, are dependent on the maintenance of and loyalty to the marginalized group. This can be viewed as healthy adaptation, a form of self-protection in response to the devaluing messages projected from the dominant group. It can also be viewed as an imprisonment because the projection of inferior status by the dominant group remains unchallenged by the culture at large. The price of marginalization is that a sense of being "other," of being less than becomes internalized. Even though there may be conscious awareness, even anger at this sense of unfairness, the internalization of underlying shame is difficult to escape.

Heather McGhee (2021) has a somewhat different take and summarizes white privilege stating, "What privilege awareness does, at its best, is reveal the systematic unfairness, and lift the blame from the victims of a corrupt system. She goes on to say, "I think at this point in our discourse—also when so many white people feel deeply unprivileged—it's more important to talk about the world we want for everyone." In other words, McGhee aims to shift the focus from what racism costs people of color to what racism costs everyone.

Molly Merson (2021) addresses the question of white privilege by asking therapists to take ownership of the impact that whiteness has had on our field, both personally and structurally. She cautions us against the suggestion that "whiteness and racist injustice can be repaired or even addressed via *mutual* recognition" (p. 17). Rather, she invites us to begin by reminding ourselves the land on which we live and work "was appropriated by willing and unwilling people, some here of their own accord, some displaced, and some enslaved in order to create prolific wealth for others" (p 18). This is a sobering reminder that can ground us and move us into spaces of greater humility.

When members of any marginalized group begin to question the ingrained assumptions or rules of socio-cultural engagement, privilege, or advancement, whether that involves family or group membership or whether it involves challenging the assumptions of the dominant group around privilege, this generally poses some form of loss, punishment, and sometimes even death. Therefore, from a clinical perspective, when treating people whose ethnic or cultural background is different from one's own, a critical aspect of our work, is to enter into a *different* relational contract, one that gives the client permission to speak up about social norms and values, to question what constitutes fairness and unfairness. Open dialogue and curiosity must come from both sides of the relational equation, which means examining unconscious biases and assumptions.

The APA points to well-established psychological principles, such as the concept of implicit bias and intergroup relations, to help guide education and training initiatives. Implicit bias and unconscious assumptions about others unlike ourselves can also be viewed as the internalization of a societally-sanctioned, collective loyalty contract. As therapists, in order to build a solid therapeutic connection, we not only need to create a holding environment that is safe, but we must also do so in a way that begins to invite curiosity and encouragement to speak into our dialogue as a way of challenging negative assumptions that may had been internalized on both sides of the therapeutic relationship.

Understanding the various historical roots and cultural variables that explain socio-cultural as well as familial loyalty contracts can increase a therapist's empathy and cultural sensitivity. A huge part of creating this new contract will involve the therapist's ever deepening understanding of power and privilege and how this shows up in the room. Dominance and submission dynamics are always at play, and they require ongoing attention. Mentioning it once or twice is not enough – think of it as the water you're both swimming in. A therapist's privileges, if unaddressed in the room, may reinforce unconscious assumptions on the part of both parties. Furthermore, it is important for therapists to have a clear formulation of the rules and assumptions contained within a patient's loyalty contract because most patients have internalized these rules and assumptions so deeply that they remain outside of conscious awareness.

When we, as therapists, clearly articulate the loyalty contract in our own minds, we can begin to engage in a dialogue with our clients in the service of increasing their curiosity about reflexive patterns and enactments. Once enactments can be articulated verbally between the therapist and client, the loyalty contract can be consciously examined, and healthier expectations of what to expect from relationships can be incorporated.

Loyalty Contracts That Create a Double Bind Message

A further way to understand the function of the loyalty contract is to see it as a parent's projection of their unfinished business that is placed onto the child. The expectations often center around a communication to either make up for the parent's disappointment by living the life they never had, or it is a message of discouragement based on fears that life will disappoint, and you can never be too careful. Often these types of loyalty contracts are confusing because they give a mixed message that conveys competitive resentment when the child succeeds as well as conveying derisive contempt when the child is not capable of living up to the parent's standards of perfectionism. The vicarious wish for the child to make up for the parent's disappointment or the competitive desire that the child not exceed and overshadow the parent creates a no-win situation for both parties. It creates a double bind that often lasts well into adulthood, because at the heart of the loyalty contract is a resistance to self-assertion and mutual recognition. When the child moves into adulthood parental control, punishment, excessive worry, or mistrust are often communicated in an effort to unconsciously maintain the expectations of the old loyalty contract through guilt or fear of loss of the relationship altogether.

An example of this double bind message that is initially communicated in childhood and then later in adulthood is as follows:

> *"If you marry a doctor, I'll feel proud of you because it proves I was a good mother and I can brag about you to my friends. If you don't marry a doctor, I'll be gravely disappointed and continue to ask you "Where did I go wrong. Was I a complete failure? I won't question whether I have a right to ask you to live out my hopes and ambitions; I have a right to expect that my life will have meaning through the visible demonstration of the success of your life, as this will be a reflection my life and who I am."*

> *And yet…*

> *"When you do marry a doctor and I see how much better your life is than mine, then I'll secretly resent you – I will see that you've left me, and that wasn't part of the bargain. Now, I'm alone and miserable, so I'll begin to overtly criticize you for other things. You won't ever be able to do anything right in my eyes. I'll try to make you feel guilty and small and miserable, so you'll end up just like me, after all."*

Dismantling Loyalty Contracts with Double Bind Messages

In this section we will explore a client example to illustrate how early attachment failures play out through the enactment of loyalty contracts which reflect double bind messages that result in a no-win situation for the client. In this client example the double bind largely stems from the mother's life-long sense of disappointment about giving up her own dreams, where she feels somehow cheated by life due to choices that she made that led to regret or frustration. Here we see the generational impact that occurs when a parent avoids taking responsibility for her own psychological issues, leaving her with chronic, though disavowed feelings of anxiety, depression, and competitive rage. Both her longings for something more as well as her negatively disavowed feelings are then projected onto her eldest child in the form of a double bind loyalty contract.

Client Example One

This is a 33-year-old woman, married with one child, who is the owner of her own successful software company. She comes from a family of privilege and describes her family of origin as being quite loving and close-knit, parents providing the patient and her sister with every opportunity in life. Patient feels closer to her father and describes mother as highly anxious, a bit over-protective, and someone who would become easily hurt if she felt slighted.

The patient's role in the family was to be the peacemaker between mother and father, as well as mother and the rest of the extended family. She took pride in this role until recently when her business took a downturn, and her mother decided to gift her the money to help with cash flow. Several months later, mother began to ask her daughter when she might be able to pay the money back. The patient was confused and told her mother that she thought that the money was a gift. Her mother quickly recanted and said, "Not to worry, you don't have to pay me back." Later in the same conversation, she asked the patient if she was spending too much time at the office and not paying enough attention to her four-year-old daughter. When the patient reported this conversation to her therapist, she stated that her mother gives her mixed messages all the time. "I know she wants me to succeed in my business, but she also has to remind me of how much she sacrificed to be a stay-at-home mom, that being a good mother is the most important thing you can give a child, and that she doesn't regret giving up her career as an opera singer to raise her two girls." These mixed messages were part of what brought this patient into therapy.

Other noteworthy patterns within the mother-daughter dyad involve the mother triangulating other family members when mother and daughter have a difference of opinion. For example, on a visit to the patient's home, her mother seemed to be particularly anxious and at one point, mother criticized the patient's husband over the upkeep of their home. She insisted on cleaning their house from top to bottom despite the patient's husband's protests. An argument then developed between mother and son-in-law, at which point mother threatened to leave abruptly. The patient became upset, trying to smooth things over by minimizing mother's behavior, which angered her husband for taking sides. The patient reported feeling caught in a double bind, having to choose with husband or mother. The patient also reported that this was not the first time that she had to become the peacemaker, and she couldn't understand why her husband couldn't let these episodes roll off his back like her father had learned to do.

Analysis

The work to be done in this case centers in part on making the parental loyalty contract explicit to enable the patient to extricate herself from the double bind. Mother's implicit message contained within the loyalty contract throughout her childhood could be articulated as follows. *"I sacrificed my life and career to be a good mother to you. Therefore, you owe me respect, and you have to make me proud by living the life I couldn't have."* This was played out by pushing her daughter into AP classes, sending her to private school and summers abroad during college. She often hovered over her daughter during school competitions or when important assignments were due, insisted that her ideas would help make the projects better. The patient remembers feeling embarrassed and undermined by this but failed to voice any resistance.

In adulthood, the loyalty contract played out by mother giving the patient money to help build her business – "I want you to have the career I never was able to have. But unconsciously I have feelings of resentment, therefore, you can't separate from me and live your own life because you owe me for my sacrifice." Mother's resentment over the patient being able to choose motherhood and a career was enacted by delivering ambivalent messages such as telling her daughter that she was spending too much time at work, thus neglecting her most important responsibility, that of being a good mother. It was also enacted by offering the gift of money but threatening to take it back, either by saying the money was a loan, not a gift, or by making veiled threats to discontinue her trust fund for reasons that remain unclear.

Once the therapist and the patient were able to clearly identify the mixed messages that resulted in the patient feeling trapped in her old role of rescuer and peacemaker, she stopped trying to lift mother out of her chronic states of depression and/or anxiety. Her initial fear that her mother would not speak to her for months if she tried to set a limit was lifted as the therapist and patient worked on ways to speak more directly to her mother about her confusion and her frustration. Rather than placating her mother by offering suggestions and solutions or being the go-between delivering messages to her father, she let her mother know that mom had some difficult choices to make and that she needed to talk with her own husband about what to do, not to use her as a mediator. In other words, the patient was able to hand the responsibility for mother's life back to her mother.

The patient was also able to speak with her own husband about future family visits, where they were able to decide together how they would set ground rules for visits and delivering those messages as a united front. This, in turn, helped curtail triangulated situations, and the patient no longer felt torn about where her new loyalties would lie. The positive outcome in this case was that the mother was able to tolerate these new boundaries; she became more contained around her daughter, and their relationship remained intact with new rules comprised of an adult-to-adult loyalty contract in place.

Identifying and Dismantling Loyalty Contracts in Couples Therapy

This section focuses on the examination of couples' communication difficulties as a reflection of unrequited longings that stem from early attachment injuries. Disappointed expectations often trigger feelings of unworthiness, mistrust, anger, and/or acts of retaliation thus revealing elements of each individual's learned loyalty contract. When misunderstanding or misattunement occurs, this becomes an unconscious trigger that activates internalized assumptions fueling the escalation of conflict or punishing withdrawal. In this section we will specifically examine how shame or mistrust become triggered by tracking the relational dynamics that become expressed within Quadrants Three and Four. We will also use the Four Quadrant Model and the Healthy Self-Actualizing Model to illustrate how defensively based reactivity can shift into healthier interaction through the understanding of patterns and triggers of each individual's loyalty contract.

The following case illustration provides insight into how a couples' enactment of their respective loyalty contracts left scars of shame and insecurity that threatened to end the marriage. Both experienced their respective partner as the "Doer" or aggressor, and themselves as the "Done To" or the victim. Feelings of hopelessness combined with criticism and/or self-protective withdrawal had been part of their relational dance for years. This client example is provided to illustrate how loyalty contracts that play out between couples over decades can be gradually dismantled, thus moving them into a more trusting, respectful, and fulfilling relational pattern.

In an attempt to understand and dismantle unhealthy loyalty contracts, the therapist began by exploring the rules of engagement within each individual's early family interactions, including:

- Issues and struggles within familial relationships around fairness, safety, control, and trust. This began to illuminate the rules of engagement of the early loyalty contract.
- Exploration then shifted to inquiry as to the parts of the self that had to be sacrificed in order to maintain a sense of safety and connection with primary caregivers.
- It was important for both individuals to verbally articulate the price they had to pay if they dared to break the family rules as well as any underlying fear they harbored.
- It was also important for each partner to act as a witness to these statements because it often opens a doorway of understanding and compassion for the wounded child within.

- By exposing this childlike vulnerability, this became a powerful opening for exploring each person's often unarticulated hopes – hopes that the partner would be able to make up for the unfairness of the early loyalty contract.

In a general sense, once early rules of engagement have been clarified, couples can then more easily recognize how old fears and relational assumptions are carried into current-day patterns and/or marital disputes. When each partner's fears and assumptions are brought more fully into conscious awareness, both are generally able to feel less personally attacked by the other. In turn, they are able to handle differences of opinion more openly, and they are more easily able to respond with empathy when their partner is being triggered.

In other words, bringing the details of the early loyalty contracts into verbal, conscious awareness in couples therapy can become a vehicle that can interrupt the repeated enactments in the present moment. Through communication and self-reflection, a new contract can be created, one that allows for support around healing past hurts and a shared partnership where new rules of engagement are created that foster mutuality, fairness, and trust. By intentionally creating a new loyalty contract between the couple, this can move them toward the Healthy Self-Actualizing Model of relational connectivity. (See Quadrant Three in the Healthy Self-Actualizing Model).

Client Example

When we enter this case discussion, Kathy and Ben have been attending couples' therapy for approximately six months. As empty nesters, they entered treatment at Kathy's urging because Kathy wasn't sure whether she wanted the marriage to continue. Ben very much wanted to make the marriage work and believed that the "minor" struggles that they had had throughout their 25-year marriage could be resolved if they spent time in therapy. Both successful professionals, the history of their relationship revealed that Kathy discovered that Ben had had a short-lived affair with a woman at work ten years earlier. She stated that her trust level never recovered; however, it should be noted that distrust had been a theme throughout their relationship, even prior to Ben's affair. Arguments often centered around the disciplining of the children, where Kathy felt that Ben was too controlling or harsh, and Ben believed that Kathy over-indulged the children, often siding with them against him so that she could be seen as the favorite parent. Kathy admitted to enjoying being the parent the children confided in but also stated that it was her role to be protective of them against Ben's anger.

Initial work within the treatment was centered on stabilizing the parental alliance, establishing clear boundaries and messages to the children around privileges, consequences, and mutual respect. As the tension between the couple dissipated around parenting struggles, they were then able to focus on communication patterns that would often trigger disappointment, frustration, shame, and withdrawal from each other. Using the Four Quadrant Model, the therapist was able to trace issues of mistrust to family-of-origin messages in Quadrant Three.

Regarding Ben's family of origin, he had a very domineering father who loved to debate and who always had to be "right." Ben's father, a college professor, often took the role of teacher/lecturer with his children. Ben learned that it was pointless to argue, and he often took a passive role, not wanting to engage in lengthy debate. However, with his children, Kathy often complained that he was just like his father, always lecturing and never knowing when to let an issue go. In terms of Quadrant Three, Ben's loyalty contract consisted of a learned belief that it's hopeless to ever try to convince his parents that he had a right to voice his opinion. Ben carried these expectations into adulthood, and when disagreements came up in the marriage, he generally capitulated to Kathy's demands. However, his buried frustration often came out through lecturing the children or spending more time away from home, either traveling for business or spending time with friends. His career was where his personal talents could shine (Quadrant One), and it was where his sense of personal worth and well-being were centered.

Kathy's family of origin involved a mother who was highly controlling, often emotionally dysregulated, cruel, and competitive. Mother presented a "perfect face" to the outside world, enough to fool Kathy's father, who never believed his children's complaints that their mother was mean and would hit them when he was at work. Mom played the victim, complaining that she gave her whole life to her children, but she looked for opportunities to shame her children when they spoke back to her or voiced an opinion other than what mother wanted to hear. Mother insisted that her children present a perfect image, and there was a great deal of pressure to perform academically as well as socially. Mother gave continual messages to Kathy that she wasn't good enough, and that no one would really ever love her because she wasn't attractive or sexy enough to keep a man.

As you can see both Kathy and Ben received messages that it was dangerous to speak up, that you couldn't win if you tried. Consequently, throughout their marriage, when either of them became disappointed, they would both retreat to their autonomous position, finding solace and a sense of pride in efforts that they were able to achieve on their own. Quadrant One became a safe place to withdraw when relational difficulties arose in Quadrant Three. Both individuals were fairly shame-sensitive and would justify their withdrawal by throwing themselves into their careers or stating that the other person didn't really understand them. They both enacted this withdrawal by punishing the other (Quadrant Four) – Ben through spending more and more time away from home and having a secret affair, and Kathy, by siding with the children against Ben.

What kept them together were the fundamental strengths in the relationship, including shared common values of hard work, pulling their own weight, and a commitment to raising happy, successful children. They both had strong senses of humor, a sense of fairness, and a circle of deep and abiding friendships. Both also had a strong commitment to family, a commitment to pursuing personal growth, a shared interest in travel, and a desire to make the marriage work.

Session Excerpt

What follows is an excerpt from a session where Kathy describes a pattern of how she gets triggered by Ben. Once triggered, the aftermath results in a combination of Kathy feeling ashamed and then blaming herself for not handling the situation more smoothly. When asked to describe the most recent incident, Kathy stated that this time it was something very minor. She and her husband had just purchased new porch furniture, and Ben suggested that they invite several of the neighbors over for dinner with social distancing in mind.

K: *When he suggested we do that, my initial response was to say, "Are you kidding? I don't feel comfortable having people over just yet." But then, that's where I begin to doubt myself and become so self-critical. In my head I say, why can't you just go along with it. You know he feels energized by being with people. He's an extrovert, and I'm an introvert. But I have just as much right not wanting to bring people to the house. And then I tell myself that I'm being a hypocrite. I go to work and run the risk of exposing my family to COVID. But on the other hand, don't I have a right to say no and let Ben know when I'm not comfortable?*

B: *Kathy's first reaction is to always say no. Every time, it's no. Then she feels guilty. She has some message in her head about being social. She tells herself "You've got to be social." I know that it comes from her mother. I think that's what makes her feel conflicted. She resented her mother for pushing her into being the life of the party. So, when I make a suggestion about getting together with folks, the old resentment of being forced to be social comes up and she takes it out on me.*

Th: *How does that happen?*

K: *At first, I turn the harshness against myself, but then later I find things to pick at Ben about. It may not have to do with the idea of having people over, but I look for things to find fault with him about.*

Th: *Are you aware that that's what you're doing? Are you aware that the initial disagreement was what makes you look for things to criticize him about later?*

K: *Not in the moment, but then when Ben calls me out on my irritability and we try to talk it through, that's when I realize what I had been doing. Then I feel*

> *horrible about myself. I don't know if we'll ever resolve this difference in temperament between us.*

Th: *Well, let's step back for a moment. I'm not sure this has to do with temperamental differences. If I understand you correctly, what seems to be the trigger is that you and Ben have a difference of opinion. What if we stopped framing it as being an introvert or extrovert, and simply focused on the fact that it's a difference of opinion. I'm wondering if that's threating in some way? You know, Kathy, your mother could never tolerate you having an opinion that differed from hers.*

K: *OH, NO! There would be hell to pay if you ever disagreed.*

Th: *I'm wondering if you're giving Ben a hard time by finding fault with him because the two of you have a difference of opinion about the social gathering?*

K: *Oh, my God. I'm treating him just like my mother treated me. How sick is that?*

Th: *Now wait a minute, let's walk through this a little more slowly. So, when Ben suggests doing something with other people, you get triggered, and then you go through this process in your mind where you list the reasons for saying yes, and why you also have a right to say no. But you keep spinning and spinning back and forth trying to figure out which is the right response. I wondering, what gets triggered when he suggests being with other people?*

K: *(Long Pause, Tears) Abandonment. My head tells me that other people are more interesting that I am. I know that sounds ridiculous, I'm selling myself short. I know he thinks I'm worthy and important. But there is this little girl in me... (Long Pause)*

Th: *Tell me about the little girl.*

K: *It has to do with my mother's message. "You have to be the life of the party or people will think you're a wall flower and they'll talk about you and make fun of you. But I just wanted to stay home and read and feel safe. Then, mom would say, "Look at you, you bookworm. You must not like people."*

> *Then, in college when I moved away from home, I did start to feel comfortable with people. I enjoyed going to a party and interacting with people. One time when I was home for spring break, I went to a neighborhood party and my mom went too. She saw me having fun and laughing and then came up to me and said with such distain in her voice, "Well, aren't you special, prancing around the room like you're the queen of the prom."*

Th: *Talk about giving you a mix message. How confusing, how awful for you.*

K: *Another memory is when I had just gotten engaged to Ben and some of my friends and the two families were going out to dinner to celebrate. I remember feeling so happy and excited, and then my mother pulled me aside before we went into the restaurant and said, "Honey, you smell." (Pause) Who would say that? Of course, I had taken a shower. Why would she do that? (Looks up) That's a mixed message too, isn't it?*

Th: No, actually, that's your mother trying to destroy your joy. It's as if she couldn't stand it if you had something she couldn't have at any given moment, like she didn't see you or consider you as a person separate from her.

K: Yes, yes. And what you said just made me think of another incident. I remember being in an airport with my mother, waiting to get on a plane, and there were these cute guys sitting next to us. My mother turns to them and makes an announcement that I had just gotten a divorce. She always did that. She'd share my personal information with anyone and everyone.

Th: You couldn't be a separate person. She felt like she owned you.

K: Yes!

Th: This leads us back to the whole topic of differences of opinion. That was not acceptable to your mother.

K: That's absolutely right. With my mother I was fighting for my soul.

Th: It was that intense for you, life and death. That's why I'm so glad you're hearing this, Ben, so that you can bear witness and understand on a deeper level how awful it was for Kathy. Hopefully, now when the two of you have a difference of opinion, and Kathy becomes triggered, you both have a conscious reference point that disagreement is a hot button, something that can set off an old reflexive response. Here's where the two of you can work to slow the conversation down, slow your reactivity down — because when Kathy gets triggered, the conversation speeds up.

B: Yes, it gets very sped up. Kathy says, "No," and I know it's going to be a fight. So, I've learned to tell myself, it's not worth it, and I just give in to whatever she wants to do.

K: And I see that he capitulates, and I'm afraid that he'll just become resentful later, which he does, and then I give in and say, "Oh sure, it's no big deal. Let's have the people over."

Th: So, what you both told me is that the way you reach a decision is not through a real agreement. You've both get triggered into your own pattern of reactivity. You give up rather than reach a healthy compromise.

B: Yeah, and what's sad is Kathy isn't really like that. She's not shy or an introvert. When she's with people, she's funny and smart.

K: Yes, once I'm with people and become engaged, that's true. But it's so exhausting to be triggered all of the time. I keep spinning in my head, and I withdraw to figure it out.

B: And then after she withdraws, she comes back and will then announce, "I've just made reservations for dinner for the four of us." And I'll say, "What? Where did that come from?" I get so confused, and it feels like she just did an about face.

Th: You didn't process the decision together.

B: And now, after this fighting and distancing, I usually don't even want to go out with friends anymore. It feels hopeless, and it's been this way our entire marriage.

Th: *Yes, but now we have more of an understanding of the pattern, and there are ways to interrupt this pattern of reactivity between the two of you.*

Both: *How?*

Th: *Kathy, when Ben makes a suggestion to have people over, are you aware in that moment you're being triggered?*

K: *Well, I don't know, sometimes yes and sometimes no.*

Th: *When you say no, and then when you notice that your mind starts spinning, that's a signal that you've been triggered.*

K: *Oh, yes, I can see that now.*

Th: *What if you said to Ben, "I think I'm being triggered right now." Rather than letting your head spin or withdrawing to try to sort it out on your own, what if you told him you're triggered, and then asked for his help? Ben, what do you think you would do if she said that to you?*

B: *I'd stop and say, "Ok let's talk it through. How can I help?" Or I'd try to get at what the source of her anxiety was.*

Th: *Ok, Kathy how would that be for you?*

K: *I think after this conversation, I'd be able to stop the spinning and try to reach out to him, rather than seeing him as the enemy.*

Th: *Great. And you also wouldn't feel so alone, having to solve a problem on your own. You'd be connected as you talk through a difference of opinion. Now let's say, you don't become consciously aware that you've been triggered, but you find yourself getting irritated with Ben, and start looking for ways to find fault with him. Ben, you would notice this behavior, correct? But rather than getting angry or frustrated, what if you tried to ask Kathy about her irritability? What if you said something like, "Did something just happen between us where you felt I cut you off or I said something that offended you?" This type of question gives you both an opportunity to pause and reflect, and hopefully, what got triggered will come into consciousness.*

K: *Yes, that would be helpful. It wouldn't feel like he was criticizing me or getting irritated back. It would feel like he was genuinely concerned about me, about us.*

Th: *So, those are a couple of ways you could interrupt the old pattern once you get triggered.*

Dismantling the Loyalty Contract

The example of this therapy exchange during the first six months of treatment led to Ben being able to decrease his frustration level with Kathy and take ownership for speaking harshly or dismissively when he felt challenged. Instead, he began to slow their communication process down, commenting on when he noticed a shift in Kathy's mood. He would ask if they could talk about what just happened if he noticed her beginning to withdraw. This created a fairly dramatic change in their communication patterns. Rather than feeling distant from one another for days if they experienced an injury, both parties are able to have a discussion that cleared the air relatively quickly. That left them feeling better about themselves and more hopeful about the relationship. With this overall shift in optimism, there was an increase in intimacy as well.

Ben was also tasked with working on not making snap decisions on his own without first consulting Kathy. As a result, Kathy felt more included and less likely to withdraw or retaliate with criticism. However, she still became triggered by fear, generally when she felt left out. Once upset, her feelings escalated further into feeling shame because she felt she should be beyond this by now. Emotional vulnerability continued to be uncomfortable for her, and as a result she would call herself weak or defective. Despite having more insight into why and how she got triggered, self-talk to try to calm herself down often didn't work.

In a later session, Kathy reported that she was still getting hooked. An example she gave involved Ben calling to let her know that he was coming home late from a business meeting. He tried calling again on the drive home, but Kathy admitted that she didn't pick up because she was angry and wanted to retaliate.

K: *As I heard the garage door open, I realized I had a burning knot in the pit of my stomach. I told myself to be calm, to be open, but I began criticizing Ben for not being careful, eating inside in a restaurant with four other people for 2 1/2 hours during Covid.*

B: *Yeah, and then I began explaining myself, justifying my actions, and then I told Kathy directly that I hated having to do that because it reminded me of being with my father.*

K: *When he said that I realized that I had put him in an old position where he had to justify himself in the face of someone who was being unreasonable. I apologized and said that I realize I was being the same way that my mother treated me when I was growing up. She always came down on me when I came home as a teenager. (Turning to the therapist) I want to create a shift inside of me and not do that. I've got to figure this out. Can you help me figure out how to stop myself?"*

At this moment in the therapy, we see that both Kathy and Ben are now able to articulate how they were each being triggered by the other based on past loyalty contracts with their respective parents. Here is a decision point in the session, where the therapist could have processed how they were being triggered and what they could say to each other that would have led to a better outcome (a problem-solving, left-brain intervention), or the therapist could have focused on what was actually triggering Kathy in the session at that moment (helping with affect regulation).

The therapist chose to direct the patient back to the burning knot in her stomach, stating that she felt that she had to explore the trauma trigger prior to moving forward toward behavioral change.

She began by asking Kathy to describe what the knot felt like, what it might represent. Kathy quickly labeled it as a fear of being vulnerable, explaining that her husband took a risk by going to the restaurant. The therapist shifted Kathy back to the fear inside of her, asking what was she afraid of?

K: *I'm afraid he would be having too good of a time, and that I would be second fiddle, not find me attractive or appealing enough. I hate that about myself. I'm better than that. Why do I have to be so insecure?*

Th: *So, let's go to your worst fear, what would happen if that were the case, if your husband found you to be second fiddle?*

K: *I don't know.*

Th: *Are you afraid he would leave you?*

K: *Yes, I guess so.*

Th: *It seems as though there is a belief that you have that is attached to the fear – Do you believe that if your husband ever has a good time without you, that means that you are less than, and he will eventually leave you?*

K: *Yes, I guess so. That's the way it was with my mother. You could be having a good time, and BAM! The other shoe would drop. She'd be yelling and screaming and criticizing me, calling me worthless.*

Th: *So, it's difficult for you to even imagine that he could have a good time, and then be glad to come home to you, a wife that he adores?*

K: *Yes. If he's having a good time with others, I automatically tell myself that I'm worthless. And I believe I'm worthless in that moment.*

B: *This is exactly what her mother did too. If she wasn't the center of attention, it made her crazy. She always had to be the center of attention.*

Th: *This may be a little different with Kathy. Kathy's mother couldn't tolerate the fact that anyone else could have air space in the room. She sucked up all the available oxygen. Your wife isn't like that. She has a loving heart and there is room for mutuality in your relationship. I think it has to do with her fears of being abandoned. When you're with her giving reassurance, she is able to believe you, tolerate her vulnerability and trust you. She's not yet able to maintain that trust when she's alone and her fear interrupts and takes over, like when you were out late at the business dinner. She can't quite give herself the reassurance – yet. Ben, it's important to see this difference. Kathy, it's important that you see this difference to. This is how you are NOT like your mother.*

B: *So, what should I do in these instances? Can I say, "I see that look on your face, that look of fear. Can you tell me what you're thinking?"*

Th: *Yes, that might work. But I wonder if that question might pull her up into her head too much. Generally, when someone is really scared, what they need is comfort. What might you do to comfort her, give her reassurance? This is how the two of you can co-regulate, much like what you would do with a small child.*

K: *I remember when our son was very little and couldn't calm down. I would sit behind him Indian style, and just hug him. That calmed him down.*

Th: *Why don't you try doing that with each other right now? (They do so, and Kathy begins to cry softly in relief).*

In the second excerpt of this case vignette, we see how working with affect-regulation in the session, first the therapist with Kathy, and then having Kathy and Ben practice with each other, became a way to use right-brain-to-right-brain interventions within the couples' session. Over time, this in turn helped them gradually let go of the repeated pattern of relational mistrust and self-protection. Witnessing each other's vulnerability as a child at the hands of controlling and/or cruel parents also increased their empathy and compassion for each other. It also enabled them to "call each other out" when old assumptions and enactments were triggered in a way that was helpful not shaming.

At the end of the therapy, the couple summarized their reflections and their work in therapy in the following excerpt.

K: *I had a chance to review all of my notes from our year and a half in therapy. What is realize is the work of healing old pain can only happen relationally. My old pattern was to tell myself, "Let me figure this out on my own, then I can come back and be ok." But you and Ben provided the safety for me to show myself when I was feeling most vulnerable and most insecure. I didn't feel attacked or unsafe.*

B: *This was certainly one of the major shifts in our relationship, in our ability to communicate with each other. I felt that I could reach you rather than having you withdraw and leave me alone and confused.*

K: *I've been pushing away from my feelings all of my life because feelings weren't safe. I'd try to intellectualize my way out of a problem. Now, I'm trying to drop into my heart, and because of our work, I've discovered that it's a much safer place to land.*

Th: *Yes, and Ben that's where you've learned how to come in and provide comfort or ask Kathy what she needs from you. You've also been able to gently reflect to Kathy when you notice her moving away without her hearing your words as a criticism. You both have been able to talk through your disagreements without either of you giving in or making decisions based on fear of upsetting the other.*

B: *Yes, and the tension level in our home is almost non-existent. We enjoy being with each other as well as having our own solo activities.*

K: *Yes, it's such a balance, coming together and moving apart. And that's still a work in progress. It's really making a choice every day – this is the person I want to be with.*

B: *And making a choice to meet up every day, whether it be cooking or taking a run together. Actually, it's been 31 years today since our first date.*

Th: *Congratulations. This is rather an auspicious day for our termination session.*

B: *You know what therapy did for me? It gave me a much greater appreciation of what it must have been like for Kathy living with her mother. Even some of the smallest details, like Kathy telling her mother that she didn't want mustard on her sandwich, and every time, her mother would put mustard on her sandwich. She didn't even accommodate to the most simple, little requests. It must have been so awful.*

K: *That's where I felt seen. Ben, when you were able to see it and understand it, that's when I realized, "Oh, my God. I'm not alone. (Long Pause) I'm tempted to just sit with this feeling… I'm not alone. (Looks up at therapist) That was one of your greatest pieces of advice – just sit with the discomfort. I'm just feeling the sadness right now.*

Th: *What's the sadness?*

K: *A sadness, but a gratefulness that I'm more in touch that that little girl. (Pause) I feel my intuition is getting stronger when I listen to that little girl. And that's where I feel more in the flow. And I didn't have that ability to listen to myself when I was growing up because I was in survival mode. And now, listening to myself, life is getting easier.*

Th: *Part of what gives us the ability to shift out of survival mode is that you've learned that you can allow yourself to listen to when you don't feel safe and then express what you need to correct that feeling state. You can't do that while you're actually in survival mode because your energy is focused on surviving in any way you can. If you allowed yourself to acknowledge how really scared you were, you may have collapsed.*

K: *Well, that just goes to show the resilience of the self, doesn't it?*

As you can see, understanding and articulating loyalty contracts within a couples' session can lead to quite powerful results. In this case the gradual dismantling of the old loyalty contracts has given way to the couple being able to tolerate increased levels of vulnerability with each other. As a result, the former enactment of withdrawal into pseudo-independence as a means of self-protection gave way to direct communication. Susan Johnson (2019), creator of Emotion Focused Therapy (EFT) states, "Attachment security predicts almost every identified indicator of positive functioning, while insecurity is a risk factor for almost every identified indicator of dysfunction" (p. 23). Understanding each individual's loyalty contract within the couples' system is one way to access underlying attachment injuries in the service of healing and repair. Much like Johnson's approach using EFT, finding ways to access and express emotional vulnerability within couple's communication patterns allows for the development of increased trust by creating relational experiences that allow for healing and repair.

It is by working with these reenactments that couples can begin to recognize repeated quid pro quo patterns that convey both their hopes and their fears. This client example provides an illustration of how conscious and unconscious triggers can be dismantled thereby allowing couples to demonstrate aspects of the Healthy Self-Actualizing Model both on an intrapsychic (Quadrant One) and interpersonal level (Quadrant Three).

Then, through understanding what triggers relational disappointment, the couple was able to dismantle their hyper-reactive triggers that created re-activity and retaliation (Quadrant Four). When that occurred, the couple was able to demonstrate improvement in communication, problem solving, and the expression of increased intimacy. This can then become inter-nalized into a healthy, self-reinforcing loop.

Chapter Summary

Loyalty contracts are a powerful force within the human psyche. The unconscious grip of a loyalty contract is conveyed by messages, expecta-tions, and values contained within the family system as well as the culture at large. The rules and values of a family system to some degree can best be understood as a reflection of the dominant culture's values and standards – the macrocosm reinforcing the microcosm, reinforcing the macrocosm, in a relatively unexamined feedback loop. There is often a huge cost to un-examined loyalty contracts. If individuals within a family system perceive that they fall short of cultural or parental expectations, a sense of shame and unworthiness becomes internalized and will often inhibit the devel-opment of a healthy, resilient sense of self. This affects both marginalized individuals, as well as people of privilege.

Relational patterns can often be more clearly understood through the framework of learned loyalty contracts. Generally, loyalty contracts are either poorly known, outside of awareness, or accepted as "this is just the way things are." Although unformulated, these automatic relational response patterns are a significant factor and a driving force in a person's life. When there is an absence of curiosity and self-reflection about something that has a pervasive significance in one's life, there is a high likelihood that unconscious power of these unresolved forces will make themselves known through repeated enactments.

We can recognize when a loyalty contract is at play by seeing the pre-dictability of patterns in the choices people make and how they repeatedly behave in relationships. Once patterns are revealed and disappointment or fear about the unfairness of the early loyalty contract have been expressed, individuals can begin to have a better grasp of the cost this has had on the self. With this comes grief and hopefully repair through the development of an earned secure attachment. As a result of this process clients are better equipped to break the grip that connects unrequited longings to early at-tachment failures. As Robert Grossmark (2016) reminds us, "Many of our most troubled patients had parents who simply could never be with them in any meaningful manner as their lives and experiences developed. When we are with these patients but do not try to do anything to them, we create the possibility of a new beginning and provide the ballast that the ensuing journey may require" (p. 294). Herein lies the power of working with loyalty contracts. It is where psychodynamic practice can operationalize the value of attachment theory through providing an environment of relational repair of the malattunement of unfair loyalty contracts.

A further examination of how to dismantle loyalty contracts will be covered in Chapter Six where the focus will be on splitting, dissociation, and part-whole analysis. Discussion of how enactments reveal a patient's internalized loyalty contract will be of further focus in Chapter Seven where we will examine how to create leverage into penetrating deeply internalized patterns that play out through the transference/counter-transference exchange.

References

Beebe, B., Jaffe, J., Markese, S., Buck, K., Chen, H. Cohen, P., Bahrick, L., Andrews, H., & Felds, S. (2010). The origins of 12-month attachment: A microanalysis of 4-month mother-infant interaction. *Attachment and Human Development*, Jan., *12*(0), 3–141.

Beebe, B., & Lachmann, F. (1988). The contribution of mother-infant mutual influence to the origins of self – and object representations. *Psychoanalytic Psychology*, *5*(4), 305–337.

Benjamin, J. (1988). *Bonds of love: Psychoanalysis, feminism, and the problem of domination.* Pantheon Books.

Benjamin, J. (2018). *Beyond doer and done to: Recognition theory, intersubjectivity and the third.* Routledge,

Ferenczi, S. (1949). Confusion of the tongues between the adults and the child (The language of tenderness and of passion). *International Journal of Psycho-Analysis*, *30*, 225–230.

Grossmark, R. (2016). Psychoanalytic companioning. *Psychoanalytic Dialogues*, *26*(6), 698–712.

Helms, J. E. (2020). *A race is a nice thing to have: A guide to being a white person or understanding the white persons in your life.* Cognella Academic Publishing.

Johnson, S. (2019). *Attachment theory in practice: Emotionally focused therapy (EFT) with individuals, couples, and families.* New York: The Guilford Press.

Kohut, H. (1977). *The restoration of the self.* International Universities Press.

Lyons-Ruth, K. (1999). The two-person unconscious: Intersubjective dialogue, enactive relational representation, and the emergence of new forms of relational organization. *Psychoanalytic Inquiry*, *19*(4), 576–617.

McGhee, H. (2021). *The sum of us: What racism costs everyone and how we can prosper together.* Penguin Random House.

Merson, M. (2021). The whiteness taboo: Interrogating whiteness in psychoanalysis. *Psychoanalytic Dialogues 31*(1), 13–27. Routledge.

Morgan, P. (Writer), Wilson, J. (Writer), & Caron, B. (Director). (2020, November 15). Fairytale (Season 4, Episode 3). [TV Series Episode] In B. Caron, M. Harrison, P. Morgan, E. Swannell, A. Thompson. *The Crown.* Left Bank Pictures and Sony Pictures Television for Netflix.

Stern, D. (1985). *The interpersonal world of the infant.* Basic Books.

Stern, D. (1989). The representation of relational patterns: Developmental considerations. In A. Sameroff and R. Emde (Eds), *Relationship disturbances in early childhood: A developmental approach,* (pp. 52–69). Basic Books.

Stern, D. B. (1997). *Unformulated experience: From dissociation to imagination in psycho-analysis*. The Analytic Press.

Tronick, E. (1989). Emotions and emotional communication in infants. *American Psychologist, 44*(2), 112–119.

Tronick, E. (2007). *The neurobehavioral and social-emotional development of infants and children*. W. W. Norton & Company.

Tronick, E., & Gold, C. M. (2020). *The power of discord: Why the ups and downs of relationships are the secret to building intimacy, resilience, and trust*. Little, Brown Spark.

Wachtel, P. (2014). Psychoanalysis and its social context. *Psychoanalytic Perspectives, 11*(1), 58–68.

Wilkerson, I. (2020). *Caste: The origins of our discontents*. Random House.

3 Recasting the Art of Case Conceptualization: Holding the Macro and the Micro Perspective Within a Cultural Context

Introduction

The *function* of a psychodynamic formulation is to provide a succinct conceptualization of a case and thereby guide the treatment plan. The *art* of case conceptualization lies in the ability to describe the client's humanity from a three-dimensional perspective. Case conceptualization as an art relies on the therapist's capacity to simultaneously hold the macro and the micro picture of any therapeutic encounter – in order to see how the past is reflected in the present, how the client's suffering leads to defensive adaptation, and how the authentic self is lying under the surface waiting to be recognized and called forward. For me, trying to capture this three-dimensional view almost seems as if I'm trying to penetrate time and space. Or, to put it another way, being able to grasp the complexity of case conceptualization is more like a holographic image rather than a flat representation, reminding me of the old biology books, where colored transparencies representing the major systems in the body were laid over one another in a way that we could visualize how the skeleton was supported by the muscular structure, that in turn encased and supported the internal organs, and how the arteries and veins fed the entire system.

The ability to describe the essential elements of treatment dynamics at any given moment in time requires holding the same level of complexity that was taught in elementary biology. Developing the ability to step back and see the big picture (macro-understanding) of repeating patterns, while also being able to zero in on nuances of language and emotional resonance moment by moment (micro-understanding), and then seeing how *all* of this is integrated into a working system, is at the heart of case conceptualization. Learning this skill set is a challenge, and once mastered, it is also what separates a good therapist from a great therapist.

The art of case conceptualization is that it helps to organize our thinking and our interventions into a framework that affects the pace and rhythm of the therapy. It is what helps us maintain appropriate boundaries around self-disclosure, as well as setting clear goals and expectations from the beginning

DOI: 10.4324/9781003120278-4

of treatment. Therapists who have been taught the art of creating a dynamic case formulation typically know how historical material connects to current patterns; they anticipate the emergence of transferential enactments, attend to process dynamics more closely, and are able to hold a big picture perspective that informs their treatment interventions. The ability to create an on-going and evolving dynamic case formulation allows therapists to pause rather than feel a pressure to respond, to understand the importance of *holding the therapeutic frame* around maintaining boundaries.

Attention to process dynamics helps the clinician attend to the patient's subjective experience. At times, therapists can get lost in the weeds with stories the client relates about present events, or details that distract from underlying conflicts and emotions. This is why pulling back to attend to the big picture is important. By pulling back, we are better able to see how defense structures play out through repeating patterns, how attachment injuries from the past have a direct impact on relational dynamics in the present. By attending to the macro-formulation of a case, we are able to more easily recognize how repeated patterns also lead to disappointed efforts that activate shame, hopelessness, or rage.

In the most basic sense, we are simply able to see more when we slow the process down. Taking a step back to reflect and review throughout the treatment process allows us to modify our initial case formulation and suspend our assumptions in order to reevaluate our original premises. It also helps to assess transference/counter-transference undercurrents more clearly, allowing us to be more informed as we move back into the micro-level of the relational exchange.

Throughout treatment we should be asking ourselves:

- What am I feeling with this client that is unique, or unsettling, or unclear?
- What else could I be doing that might improve or deepen the therapeutic relationship?
- How might I incorporate other treatment modalities or think about the neuro-physiological reflexive responses of my patients and respond from a position that activates right-brain-to-right-brain communication?
- What cultural variables may have impacted the client's opportunity to equal access and how might these variables play into their current struggles and symptoms?

It is this on-going curiosity that allows us to develop a more complete picture of our clients and thus keep the treatment process alive and fresh. Above all else, the power of writing a good case formulation lies in the spirit of describing a picture that captures our patient's humanity – their pain and suffering as well as their strengths, resilience, and potential.

Historical Elements of the Traditional Psychodynamic Formulation

In the past two decades we have seen a gradual shift from a medical/ mechanistic model to a more wholistic construct of the human being. The catalyst for this paradigm shift comes from the confluence of several areas of research; a.) the mapping of the genome, b.) the ability to observe a functioning brain with magnetic imaging, and c.) an increased understanding of the central nervous system based on the polyvagal theory. In addition, advances in infant research have directed our theoretical orientation toward parent/infant attachment dynamics and the importance of emotional regulation in healthy self-development. These relatively recent scientific and theoretical constructs pertaining to how people develop and function have advanced our understanding of the impact of neurophysiology, epigenetics, and the importance of culture and context on human behavioral response patterns, symptoms, and character development.

Richard Summers (2003) describes the challenge that is presented when trying to capture the complexity of a case formulation in terms of which model or template to follow. He states, "Most clinicians are in favor of the biopsychosocial model, yet this 'big tent' of psychiatric conceptualization all too often results in a bland picture lacking in depth. On the one hand, the typical biopsychosocial formulation includes a descriptive diagnosis that refers to psychological and social issues, but is lacking in inference about psychological motivation to the extent that it does not provide an adequate guide for treatment. One the other hand, the classical psychodynamic formulation provides a refined and focused picture, but is seen as antiquated and not in keeping with the remarkable developments in neuroscience" (p. 39).

Whatever model one chooses, Wilma Bucci (2011) offers clear guidance on the importance of maintaining a compassionate attitude when describing our patients' suffering, and she reminds us, "The presenting problems that bring patients to treatment – the addictions, the isolation, the self-destructive behaviors, the somatic symptoms – reflect the strategies of management of the painful affect that the person devised in earlier times, the best they could do in situations that were experienced as dangerous or even catastrophic. The strategies are not working now and are themselves problems, but the dangers are still registered in the schema and must be dealt with" (p. 220). It is in this spirit that the value of psychodynamic case conceptualization must be held.

In this next section, a brief review of the history of psychodynamic case formulation is provided to illustrate how perspectives and measures used to treat psychopathology at any given time is *based upon* as well as *limited by* a therapist's theoretical assumptions. As the trajectory of theoretical and scientific advances change, there must be a concomitant change that is reflected in how we reshape our thinking around case formulation. A brief review of psychodynamic formulation follows.

According to Friedman and Lister (1987), psychodynamic formulation was created as a teaching tool that emerged out of psychoanalytic training institutes. Later, dynamic formulations were adapted for the use of short-term psychodynamic therapy models as well. There are numerous resources on how to conduct an initial assessment interview and explicate the differential diagnosis of personality disorders, which will not be reviewed in this chapter. They include, Akhtar, 1992; Benjamin, 1993; Josephs, 1992; Johnson, 1994; Kernberg, 1984, MacKinnon & Michels, 1971; Millon, 1981; and Othmer & Othmer, 1989.

Perry et al. (1987) summarized the basic format used for most traditional psychodynamic formulations. The four essential elements of a formulation include: (i) *a general summary of the case*, including identifying information, precipitating events, quality of interpersonal relationships, and salient past history, (ii) *a description of non-dynamic factors*, including genetic predisposition, trauma, deprivation, and substance abuse, (iii) *a description of core, central conflicts*, which trace central conflicts through personal history, adaptive and mal-adaptive attempts to resolve conflict on the part of the patient, identification of conscious and unconscious wishes, motives, behaviors, and defenses, and important developmental struggles, (iv) *a prognostic assessment of the course of treatment*, identifying potential areas of resistance, a patient' experience of prior treatment, and probable transference manifestations.

McWilliams (1999) expanded the scope of case conceptualization from diagnosis and prognostic outcome of treatment to a focus on process dynamics and to turn that into "a narrative that makes this human being and his or her psychopathology comprehensible to us" (p. 76). She also stated that the central diagnostic task of a clinical interview is to assess the developmental level of the person's character organization. Mc Williams' broad assessment of how a client is organized characterologically was divided into three categories – symbiotic-psychotic, borderline, or neurotic. Additionally, she suggested the applicability of the type of treatment recommended – (1) supportive therapy, (2) expressive therapy, and (3) uncovering therapy, respectively, which were based on patients with these differing character structures. Finally, she added new categorizations of data into the traditional formulation, which include temperamental and organic factors as well as identifying the individual's sense of "personhood," sexual orientation, affect regulation and reality testing.

Goldman and Greenberg (2015) developed a case formulation framework based on Emotion-Focused Therapy (EFT). Their framework, similar to Nancy McWilliams, focuses primarily on the clients' narrative content. However, their main emphasis is on identifying the client's emotional processing style, including affective meaning states, non-verbal expression, emotional arousal vs emotional productivity, the client's capacity to regulate his/her emotional experience, all of which is understood within the context of the client's early attachment history. The organization of the case formulation analysis is based on assessing the patient's emotional processing style and how one's sense of self and core pain is connected to "problematic emotion schemes that are emblematic of problematic affective-meaning states that are in need of transformation or repair through the therapeutic process" (p. 17). The task of the therapist is to formulate "markers" that track themes, identify triggers and behavioral consequences of the underlying, problematic emotion schemes. Markers provide for the therapist ways of identifying particular types of affective problems that lead to dysfunctional processing in the service of facilitating resolution of various types of processing problems (Elliott et al., 2004; Greenberg et al., 1993; Rice & Greenberg, 1984).

The concept of schemas is not a new one. Wilma Bucci (2011) talked about emotion schemas as a way to understand and describe how people experience themselves in relation to others, what they expect from life and relationships, how feeling states are regulated and processed, and how individuals develop strategies for living. Stolorow et al. (1987) and later Orange et al. (1997) referred to the term organizing principles, called "affective schemas," in a similar fashion, which grows out of the child-caretaker system of mutual interaction, where recurring, repeated patterns of the intersubjective interaction during development give rise to principles that unconsciously organize later adult experiences. Also referred to as internal maps, these schemas are part of what comprise an individual's self-concept as well as expectations and patterns within adult relationships. Bucci expands on the concept of schemas and connects emotion schemas to multiple code theory and neuronal processing, stating that the human organism is a "multi-state, multi-format information processors. She states that if we are able to identify basic psychological processes associated with changes in emotion schemas, this assessment strategy can be applied across various schools of psychotherapy practice.

Approaches to Assist in Macro-Understanding of Case Formulation

Often, students will ask, "How do you even begin to think about choosing what pieces of information are important about a case? Which details are relevant, and which ones can be eliminated from the case formulation write-up? How can you hold the various components and/or dynamics of a case in your mind at the same time?" These are important questions when it comes to understanding the macro-level of case formulation.

In this section, two representations of how to hold or capture the macro-formulation of a case will be presented. The first lists six broad categories of inquiry, with detailed questions listed within each category, to help capture the unique qualities of individual patients. The second schematic represents a macro-view of a case by providing, 1.) a visual graphic that depicts the relationship between quality of early attachments, 2.) level of stability of affect regulation, and 3.) degree of shame sensitivity. Seeing the relationship between these three variables in action will result in a better understanding of how defensive organizing systems are constructed.

The list provided below offers a series of six categories that will help identify a macro-picture of case conceptualization. Key areas for reflection will; a.) connect past to present, b.) connect underlying beliefs to current behaviors, and c.) connect expectations of self and other to symptoms, longings, and the degrees of reactivity. The bullet point items beneath each major category are meant to provide a more detailed picture of the patient's organizing schemas. Understanding as many details as possible contained within each category enables the therapist to gain a more complete picture of the complexity of the client's specific organizing schemas.

I   **Look for Patterns** – How do you determine if something is a pattern?

- Is there enough data to show a repetition in thoughts, beliefs, or behaviors over time?
- What degree of insight does the patient possess with regard to repeating behavioral patterns?
- Does the patient retain a congruent and sustained memory of entering into the same potentially dangerous or unrealistic situation – or does s/he have little or no ability to recognize red flags?
- Does the patient use "justifications" saying that this time things will be different?

Note: Repeated dysfunctional patterns are generally based on beliefs or behaviors that are not well-grounded in reality but represent unconsciously driven fantasies or unrequited wishes and longings from childhood.

II   **Look for Beliefs about Self and Other**

- What do they expect from themselves?
- What do they expect from others? Is what they expect from others different from expectations of self?
- How do they feel about receiving help, trusting others, relinquishing control?
- How do they handle disappointments in life?

  - Is there a sense of harshness, cynicism toward self or others?
  - Do they tend to excuse bad behavior on the part of self or others?

III **Family of Origin** – Look for the Quality of Early Attachment.

- Do they overly idealize their caretakers?

- What are their relational expectations around trusting others?
- Are their relational expectations realistic, over-idealized, cynical/ defeatist?
- Are they able to consciously *articulate* what they expect from others?
- Are they passively waiting for rescue from another?
- Do they overly excuse or overly blame others when they are hurt, disappointed or treated unfairly?
- What is their stance toward commitment, mutuality, transparency in relationship?

IV How Does the Person Approach/Negotiate Life

- How successful is s/he in achieving goals and at what cost?
- Does the person display aspects of spontaneity, joy, playfulness, humor?
- Is there a high degree of reactivity/impulsivity, or do they have a sense of purpose and capacity for follow-through?
- Does the person adopt a position of passivity, sense of fatalism, or does s/he expend overly-determined efforts to achieve goals?
- What is their performance measure for accomplishment – perfectionistic/realistic?

V Is the Presenting Issue Situational or Chronic?

- Why is this particular external stressor throwing the patient off balance at this time?
- If an external stressor doesn't seem to be present, how does the patient understand why the symptoms are occurring?
- What is the patient willing to do with regard to lifestyle changes to help ameliorate the symptoms?

Note: How you answer these question helps with setting treatment goals. It also helps to determine the timing and the pace of interventions.

VI Assess for Shame Sensitivity: Degree of Over-Compensation – (What is being hidden from the therapist, what is unconscious or disavowed within the patient).

- Is s/he aware, but embarrassed to reveal emotional vulnerability or the need for help?
- When triggered by shame, can the patient consciously register the feeling and the trigger, or is there an immediate move to reflexively blaming others or conversely to criticizing the self?
- When triggered by shame, does the patient become dissociative, unable to access feelings or is s/he able to stay in the present moment?

- How might the patient's feelings of shame be connected to early attachment failures?
- What is the patient's general level of trust in others, trust in the therapeutic process?

Note: This will forecast how solid the therapeutic relationship can become, how much control the patient needs to maintain, and how transferential enactments may unfold.

These six areas of focus will help you begin to conceptualize a big picture formulation of a case. The questions are aimed as assessing learned attachment patterns and expectations as well as degrees of attachment injury. Assessing the level of rigidity and fragility within the patient will help guide your thinking around setting treatment goals and monitoring the pace of treatment. Each of these six areas of focus also lend themselves to working with the Four Quadrant Model and Healthy Self-Actualizing Model.

A second way of assessing the macro-view of a case is provided in the visual graphic of Figure 3.1. This graphic captures the level of a patient's health/fragility by seeing the relationship between: capacity for self-regulation, the degree of attachment injury, and the degree of shame sensitivity. Assessing levels of rigidity and flexibility within the personality will in turn help the therapist identify the degree of defensive over-compensation that is required to maintain psychic equilibrium.

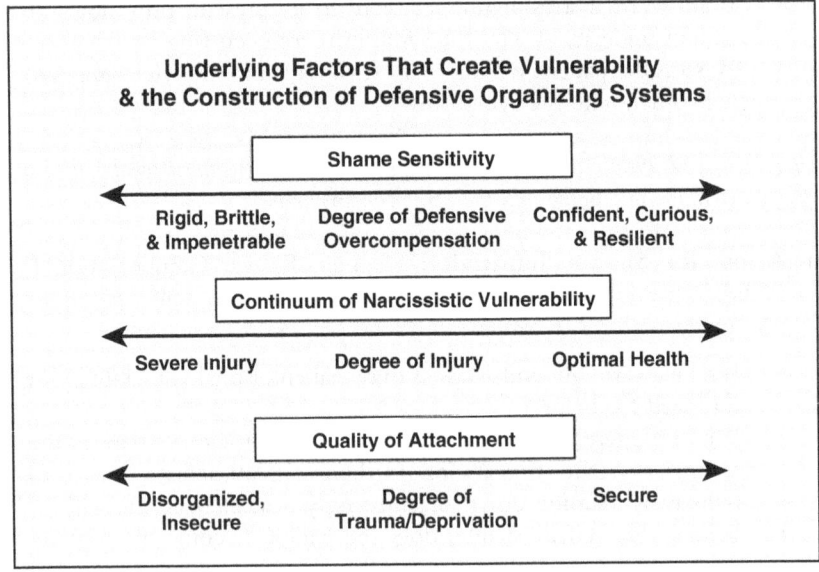

Figure 3.1 Underlying Factors that Create Vulnerability.

Entering into any of the three levels of this graphic will help you connect past history to present dynamics and symptom formation. Looking at the graphic in its entirety will help you forecast where the patient is likely to fall on the assessment continuum in terms of the balance between strengths/areas of resilience vs. the severity of the defensively driven character structure. As you refer to the Healthy Self-Actualizing Model, you can also begin to identify the areas of life where they show signs of health, pockets of resilience, spontaneity, or situational contexts where symptoms do not seem to be triggered. You would then connect these questions and observations to the quality of their early attachment. The more secure the attachment, the less psychic injury and less shame sensitivity lies under the surface. The more disorganized or insecure the attachment, the more compulsivity and over-determination will be evidenced in the defensive over-compensations around beliefs, behaviors, and attempts of keeping feelings of shame and inadequacy from breaking into consciousness. On the third line, the degree of shame sensitivity is directly correlated to the quality of early attachment, as well as to underlying feelings of vulnerability. Each of these will determine how brittle or impenetrable the defense structure is.

Incorporating Psychodynamic Formulation Schematics into Trauma Treatment

Neurophysiological advances have impacted our understanding of how we measure adaptive vs. maladaptive defense mechanisms. Trauma creates alterations in the body as well as the brain, which in turn affect capacities around affect regulation and how individuals form relationships. Neural networks in the brain are formed without the person's conscious awareness, affecting the individual's capacity to avoid or prepare for danger. Chronic trauma reduces the individual's capacity for self-reflection and self-awareness. With securely attached individuals, the naturally emergent, developmental capacities of the brain lean toward self-regulation and self-organization. However, in those individuals with insecure attachment histories, their developmental capacities lean toward avoiding danger and seeking safety; thus, they are left at a disadvantage in terms of measures that reflect affect regulation, personal ambitions, and resilience.

Formulating a differential diagnosis requires the ability to make a distinction between individuals with a single episode trauma vs. individuals who suffered from complex trauma, as defined by unsafe environments where prolonged, repeated abuse and/or neglect were interpersonally bound, leaving the child little or no chance of escape. These distinctions have implications for goal setting, course of treatment, as well as prognosis. It is important to reflect upon the individual's environment with regard to single event traumas that may or may not occur in the context of a family life that was fraught with instability when making this differential assessment. Here is where using a relationally based approach, grounded in attachment theory is useful in terms of how we redefine pathological limitations as well as how we view behavior as resistance vs. early protective survival strategies.

Unstable or depriving environments in childhood change how the brain develops or fails to develop. Unsafe environments force children into directing their energy toward safety-seeking measures. They have no choice. It is simply the result of neurobiological adaptation to that which is perceived as a threat in the environment. Brain maturation is experience-dependent. Survival efforts always take precedence, which means that the normal development of the *learning and striving brain* becomes compromised and limited where situations of chronic deprivation or lack of safety are allowed to exist. When energy is redirected toward safety, and survival preoccupies and interferes with the child's growing brain throughout developmental stages, many of the brain's capacities around regulation and soothing will atrophy while areas of the brain dedicated to maintaining safety become overly stimulated and activated. If we consider the neurobiological impact on self-regulatory capacities using right-brain-to-right-brain assessment measures, this helps us understand how the brain becomes compromised in development.

Robert Stolorow (2013) brings advances in our neurological understanding of trauma into his view of case conceptualization as well as treatment. He states: "Developmental trauma originates within a formative intersubjective context whose central feature is malattunement to painful affect—a breakdown of the child-caregiver interaffective system, leading to the child's loss of affect-integrating capacity and thereby to an unbearable, overwhelmed, disorganized state. Painful or frightening affect becomes traumatic when the attunement that the child needs to assist in its tolerance and integration is profoundly absent" (p. 385).

Allan Schore focuses on a paradigm shift from attachment theory to regulation theory which recognizes that infant brain development, including genetic coding, is the direct result of the early emotional environment comprised of the interactions between caregiver and infant, profoundly important in the first two and a half years of life. This relationship is communicated through right-brain-to-right-brain attunement between the dyad and directly impacts the neurological development of the child's brain systems including those involved in affect arousal, self-regulation, the psychic structure, and the sense of self (Schore & Schore, 2008). Combining an integrative theory of neurobiology and psychodynamic practices with attachment/regulation theory, Schore links our understanding of how trauma and severe neglect affect brain development, influencing every aspect of experience from how we perceive external stimuli as threatening or safe to one's relationship to bodily based emotions, i.e., capacities to tolerate and regulate feelings. Schore concludes that all psychological "pathologies" include difficulty with affect regulation. Therefore, treatment of attachment and self-regulation disorders must include right-brain-to-right-brain interventions.

When we assess behavioral patterns in adulthood, our challenge is to recognize how maladaptive coping strategies are attempts at regulation and stabilization. Viewing presenting problems through a neurobiological lens gives us a window into understanding the degree of traumatic injury and how we should intervene into the treatment of the trauma. Current infant research is pointing to the impact of attachment/regulation and lack of attunements as it correlates to dissociative behaviors in adolescence (Lyons-Ruth et al, 2006). A contemporary psychodynamic formulation that incorporates an understanding of how the brain has been changed and limited during critical early development due to attachment failures allows us to design a treatment plan using appropriate interventions that will mirror and attune to the client accurately. Where there is a history of trauma and/or abuse, both Schore and Stolorow stress the importance of the therapeutic relationship as a critical reparative element.

Incorporating Culture and Context into Psychodynamic Formulations Using the Four Quadrant Model

Think of the Four Quadrant Model as a pond, a pond that is constructed to protect the self from feelings of shame. When shame gets activated, it is as if a pebble has been thrown into the middle of a pond, rippling out and hitting all four quadrants. Our task as therapists is to track how the ripple effect of shame impacts the person's sense of self, relational expectations, disappointments, and symptom breakthrough. Depending on the degree of attachment injury and shame sensitivity, self-protective mechanisms will be activated. People who have mild to moderate degrees of attachment injury have a greater capacity for emotional regulation, and there will be less activation that shame triggers will have on the person's sense of stability and well-being. The greater the attachment injury, when a pebble of shame is dropped into the pond, it is more likely that shame triggers will overwhelm the individual and create hyperarousal or shutdown as well as defensive over-compensations. Therefore, when shame is activated, it will impact all of the quadrants more pervasively than in the person who has achieved a healthier sense of self as illustrated in the Healthy Self-Actualizing Model.

A historical blind spot in the creation of our psychodynamic theoretical constructs, however, (one that impacts the treatment relationship to date) has been the assumption that we all grew up in the same pond, with similar developmental challenges and opportunities more or less. *There is nothing further from the truth.* The impact of cultural marginalization around variables of race, class, gender, age, and sexual identity challenge theoretical assumptions, albeit blind spots, based on a Eurocentric lens that has the power to name and define what is viewed as normal vs. pathological. For example, assumptions remain largely unquestioned around standards that value competition, power and domination, the individual over the collective, and privilege and material consumption as measures of success, thus maintaining a social hierarchy that has yet to be effectively questioned much less challenged. Structures centered on domination and subordination require that a sub-group be devalued, treated with suspicion or contempt, seen as 'the other'.

Being treated as 'the other' produces internalized feelings of shame, self-doubt, and fear, all of which are continually culturally reinforced. Shame becomes internalized through systemically controlled access to opportunity as well as biased mythology, thus shaping the subordinated groups degree of trust, hope, frustration, opportunity, and sense of self. Conceived as inferior, including being devoid of the most basic human dignity, is then coupled with being denied the means to obtain what is valued by the culture. In turn, lack of "success" becomes the dominant cultures' proof of inferiority, lack of humanity, and rationalization for the accuracy of this destructive and demoralizing paradigm.

Paul Wachtel (2014) states, "It is quite possible to recast psychoanalytic formulation in ways that continue to address the unconscious dynamics traditionally of psychoanalytic concern and yet are simultaneously attentive to the actualities of race, class, poverty, or the myriad of daily realities that occupy center stage in most other theories of human behavior" (p. 204). And yet, the bulk of psychological theory has been shaped by white, Eurocentric influence, leaving unchallenged potential blind-spots that power and privilege have had in shaping how we view what is normal vs. pathological. The value of individualism as a cardinal feature of health as measured by the separation/individuation process, our notions around what constitutes consistent caregiving in terms of creating a secure attachment bond, even the structure and access to treatment are normed on white, heterosexual, middle class standards that have shaped both our clinical assumptions as well as intervention strategies.

For nearly a century, resources and communal values within other ethnic traditions have been undervalued or misunderstood when measured against traditional Eurocentric standards. As clinicians the very real lack of equal access for people of color, coupled with the long-term effect of internalized oppression, fear around lack of equal protection on our streets and within the legal system, are variables that we can no longer afford to overlook. Wachtel (2014) further states that the field of psychology could be of great value, providing guidance for people in terms of how to *think about* the inequalities and injustices in our society if we can better understand the anxieties, conflicts, and defenses that are differentially induced in the privileged and the less privileged by our inequalities (p. 201).

Toward that end, a recast of classical psychodynamic formulation models need to include the following:

- Understanding how blind spots around cultural norms across race and class have likely skewed our perceptions toward a dominant Eurocentric view, thus narrowing our focus around important factors of inequality and disenfranchisement that have an impact on one's sense of self, sense of place, and resilience.

• Valuing the difference around cultural norms that include: expectations around attachment and obligation to family, cultural norms around privacy, self-disclosure, and shame sensitivity, expectations around gender norms and roles.

• Weighing the impact that the dominant culture's devaluing and subordination of a particular race or ethnicity has had on a person's sense of safety, visibility, confidence, access to opportunity, resentment, powerlessness, and/or rage.

In summary, understanding the differential impact that contextual variables such as privilege and marginalization have on our clients, as well as integrating the neurobiological insights into attachment/regulation theory, and incorporating advances in trauma treatment are all critically important components that go into writing an integrated, culturally relevant case formulation. Our ability to conceptualize and craft a psychodynamic case formulation is colored by what we are able to see or not see, much of which is based on our theoretical orientation as well as our own cultural biases. Designing a case formulation that challenges potential blind spots and clinical assumptions is important in terms of holding a neutral as well as expansive view of what constitutes health and pathology. Each of the above-mentioned areas will be included in the next section as we integrate socio-cultural and neurological components into a case formulation write up using the Four Quadrant Model.

Case Conceptualization Using the Four Quadrant Model

As is the case with most case formulation models, the goal of case formulation using the Four Quadrant Model is to provide an integrated snapshot that links key developmental and relational factors to the patient's current life situation and presenting complaints. A description of the client's core conflicts will be highlighted through the identification of repeated patterns, areas of ambivalence, and/or affective triggers that generate negative emotional states. Additionally, the dynamic formulation articulates early prognostic indicators around how the treatment will unfold, including consideration of past therapeutic treatments, transferential enactments, degree of underlying shame, as well as strengths, resources, social supports, and socio-cultural considerations that may impact the case.

Most programs that teach psychodynamic formulation as a part of their training use a particular theoretical framework as a way of grounding their observations within the case formulation write-up. For example, a case formulation written by a classically trained analyst would connect presenting symptoms and patient observations to unresolved oedipal issues, areas of aggression, passivity, and fixations at the various developmental stages – oral, anal, and phallic oedipal. An object relations therapist would organize his/her observations through the lens of pre-oedipal and oedipal fixations, including the articulation of the patients' unconscious fantasies, and how the client was able to negotiate the developmental phases of rapprochement and separation/individuation. A self-psychological orientation would capture observations and symptoms through the lens of self-object functions, developmental stage of narcissistic injury, and shame sensitivity with regard to developing defense mechanisms of false self/real self.

Case conceptualization using the Four Quadrant Model is specifically designed to allow therapists from psychodynamic and non-psychodynamic orientations to apply their own theoretical approach to the design of the formulation. Although specific sections of the Psychodynamic Formulation Template draw upon attachment theory, the design of the formulation is intentionally geared toward *not being theory bound*, in hopes that the model and approach can more easily be applied across theoretical disciplines. Using an "experience-near" stance (listening to what the client is telling us in the present moment) helps us organize a picture of the client's psyche. For example, issues and concerns about the self will be placed in Quadrant One. Symptomatic complaints will be placed in Quadrant Two. Content disclosure pertaining to relational issues, wishes, complaints will be placed in Quadrant Three. How a patient expresses and handles disappointment will be placed in Quadrant Four. Furthermore, defensive over-compensations within each quadrant help in assessing the degree of shame that is under the surface of the Character Solution.

Once a picture of each of the quadrants is complete, the formulation will further assess whether parts are disconnected/split off from other parts and the whole, or where there are degrees of integration between parts of the self that comprise the client's narrative. The utility of using the visual matrix of the Four Quadrant grid is that we can more easily see where dissociative splits are occurring. This is done by tracking which quadrants are minimized by the patient, how the patient describes his or her life narrative, and factors that determine the patient's decision-making process. Finally, the Four Quadrant Model illustrates the relationship between one's individual aspirations as they are connected to relational expectations, as they are connected or disconnected from symptom break-through, and how one handles disappointments within self and within relationships.

Expanding the Understanding of the Four Quadrant Model: Questions to Help the Inquiry Process

The questions contained in this section are provided to help you delve more deeply into understanding how to use the Four Quadrant Model as an assessment tool. The more detailed the inquiry process, the more aspects of the dynamic picture are revealed. The more parts that are revealed, the more accurate your psychodynamic formulation. Remember, the Four Quadrant Model, unlike the Healthy Self-Actualizing Model, is a picture of *defensive overcompensation*. Understanding how the defense structure operates will help guide both our goal setting and treatment process.

As you study the Four Quadrant Model (Figure 3.2), you will see behaviors, beliefs, assumptions, and coping attempts to achieve a sense of homeostatic stability.

The list of questions provided below are designed to help you anticipate and listen for what might organically come up within any given session over time. By starting at a *Micro-level*, these questions actually help to capture the *Macro-view of case conceptualization*. The particular questions placed in each respective quadrant are meant to help you apply the organization of the Four Quadrant Model and the Healthy Self-Actualizing Model into the actual therapeutic inquiry process throughout the treatment relationship. These questions can also assist in better identifying what is initially hidden from the treatment relationship. Because various components of each quadrant will be revealed over time, the questions also provide guidance as

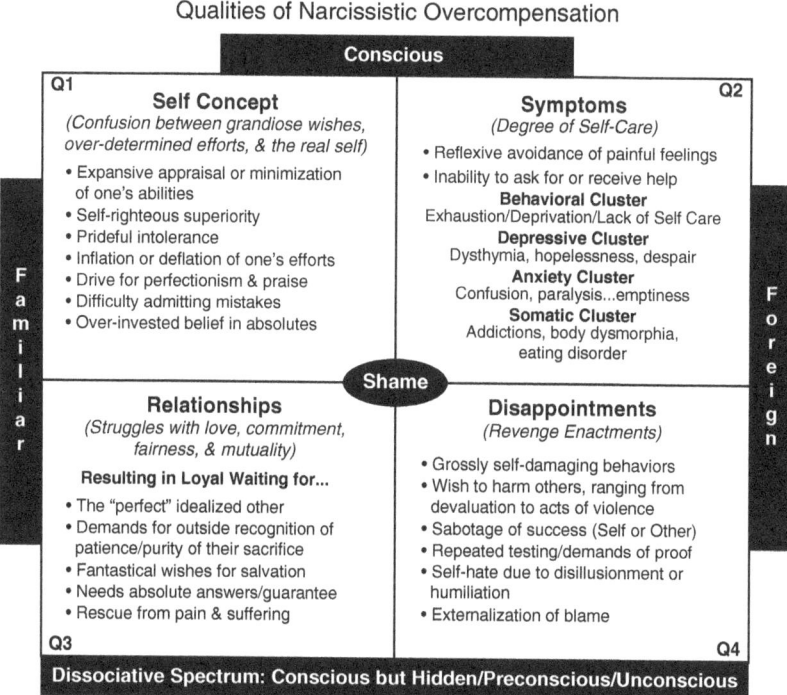

Figure 3.2 The Four Quadrant Model.

to what you might ask as follow up inquiry after the initial assessment phase of treatment. The questions in italics are provided as a means of expanding your thinking around factors that pertain to potential factors around cultural marginalization as it might impact each of the four quadrants.

Questions That Pertain to Quadrant One

1 **How would clients describe who they are and what is important to them?** *What are your client's relevant social identities? What do these identities mean to them? If white, what is their awareness of privilege and their relationship to privilege? For people of color, do they acknowledge their "difference" in terms of being proud, or do they internalize the messages of society that says they're less than?*

2 **What do they expect of themselves in terms of performance, ambition, dreams?** *In light of potentially negative internalized social identities, what did they learn about how they should perform, what they should strive for, and what their dreams should be?*

3 **What kind of standards do they have with regard to self? Are they kind, forgiving, harsh, curious, open, rigid?** *How much of their standards with regard to self are based on what they've internalized from the standards of the society?*

4 **What is the level of self-reflective capacities with regard to these standards?** *For those persons who are not self-reflective, to what extent is their lack of self-reflection a defensive stance of protection due to experiencing themselves as a marginalized or privileged person?*

5 **How do they interpret the world – do they rush to judgment or can they process and accommodate new information into their narrative?** *More specifically, if they are white, how much are they showing evidence of internalized white superiority (individualism, "professionalism," expectation of comfort, self-congratulations, arrogance/expertism, and more)? If they are BIPOC, how much are they showing evidence of internalized racial inferiority?*

6 **How does the client experience making a mistake or falling short of a goal?** *If they belong to a marginalized group, what additional costs do they bear for making a mistake or falling short of a goal due to being a member of their group(s)? If a member of a privileged group, do they have expectations that their privilege will protect them?*

7 **Do they hold the same standards toward self as they do for others? If different, why?**

8 **What is their relationship to their own feelings?**

    • are they aware of their feelings?
    • do they choose to show their feelings, do they suppress their feelings?
    • can they integrate evidence/cognitions into their feelings?

- how are feelings linked to responses?
- is there variability or is there a consistent pattern?

9 **How do they present themselves to others?**

- easy confidence,
- over-confident (grandiose),
- unsure, always questioning self.

10 **Do they hold a realistic picture of their own limitations and accept these limitations – what core insecurities may initially be hidden from view, what is their degree of shame sensitivity, to what extent do they try to avoid experiencing feelings of shame or feeling less than?** *To what extent are they (or you) aware of how sociocultural conditioning affects how they view their limitations, their core insecurities, their shame sensitivity? To what extent do they try to avoid experiencing feelings of shame or feeling less than?*

Questions That Pertain to Quadrant Two

1 **What is their degree of self-awareness with regard to how they approach life and their symptoms?** *How does their sociocultural conditioning impact how they view the relationship between how they approach life and their symptoms?*

2 **How much shame is attached to having symptom breakthrough?**

3 **What approaches have they used in the past to ameliorate symptoms?**

4 **What wishes do they bring to you with regard being able to help with symptom relief?** *Are there areas of guardedness or suspicion that they harbor around receiving help or symptom relief that might make sense based on their sociocultural context and lived experience?*

5 **Do they expect a quick resolution, or are they willing to work on getting to the root cause of the symptom?** *Based on their lived experience as a privileged or marginalized person, can their life outside support this more intensive work?*

6 **What degree of self-medication is being used to manage or distract from symptoms?**

7 **Are they willing to change behaviors that may be causing the symptoms, or are they expecting some magical cure?**

8 **What is their stance on taking medication – assess level of resistance/shame.** *What are the sociocultural influences on their view of medication?*

9 **What is their history in terms of genetic vulnerabilities or other medical issues that may be contributing to symptoms?**

10 **When is the last time that they have had a physical, thyroid test, other medical tests that should be used as a rule-out for presenting symptoms in treatment?** *If they belong to a marginalized group, what is the quality of their medical care? If they are transgender or nonbinary, do they even have access to gender affirmative medical care?*

Questions That Pertain to Quadrant Three

1 **What do they expect from an intimate relationship – from friendships?**
2 **How much do they trust others – blind trust, guarded, overly self-reliant, paranoid?** *Explore how these reactions to trust make sense in light of their social identity.*
3 **To what extent do they actually get to*know*the person before jumping into a relationship?**
4 **How do they ascertain whether someone can actually meet their needs?** *With their sociocultural conditioning and context in mind, what is their attitude toward personal needs separate from the group needs? If group needs are paramount, is there a cost? What individual needs are paramount, what are the costs?*
5 **What are their wishes in terms of being in a relationship, what do they long for?**
6 **Is their desire to be in a relationship based on an accurate assessment of the other, or is the connection based on fantasy/ longing?**
7 **What are their expectations of others in terms of mutuality and fairness?** *If they belong to a marginalized group, how has a subordinated status influenced how they should be treated by 1) more powerful others 2) equally powerful others 3) less powerful others?*
8 **When dysfunctional relational patterns are repeatedly re-enacted, what is the client's level of conscious awareness of these patterns?** *How much awareness is there about the impact of their sociocultural conditioning on problematic relational patterns?*
9 **What is their reaction if/when you point out the possibility of the pattern to them – do they minimize, do they feel increased shame, do they dissociate?** *If you hold a more powerful social identity than your client, how does that influence what occurs between you when you point out problematic patterns?*
10 **Do they make excuses for a partner or parent's bad behavior, or do they become reactive and jump to criticism and mistrust, or do they go back and forth?** *If they make excuses, how might their marginalized status **or** highly privileged status influence this?*

Questions That Pertain to Quadrant Four

1 **How do they react to disappointment?** *Thinking about the influence of a trauma history (epigenetics), how might these experiences influence how the client reacts to disappointment?*

2 **Do they integrate disappointment with others into long-term memory, or does it disappear when a person comes back into the picture making promises?** *How might this be a way for a traumatized/marginalized person to manage their internalized oppression? How might this be a way for a traumatized/marginalized person to maintain connection with someone who holds more social and economic power?*

3 **Do they retaliate or hold onto a grudge?**

4 **Can they discern different levels of disappointment or do all disappointments hold the same weight?**

5 **How do they react when disappointed in themselves?** *Does their internalized oppression or privilege show up in the form of aggression toward self, or is it projected onto others?*

6 **Does it trigger shame, does awareness of shame create more shame, or do they minimize their responsibility and blame others?** *Are they more prone to self-criticism based on their marginalized status (e.g. a black woman is disappointed by a lower than expected performance review at work but doesn't seek clarification about what she suspects are unfair ratings; she then concludes that she should have worked harder despite putting in more hours and effort than her peers)? Or, are they prone to minimize responsibility and blame others based on harm inflicted due to their marginalized status (e.g. a woman with a disability, compromised mobility, is unable to attend her friend's wedding due to poor accessibility offered, interprets this as not caring about her.)*

7 **Do they lash out – either against self or others?** *How might this be an expression of their internalized oppression? Do they collapse under the weight of self-criticism based on their identity? Or, do they regulate their shame by shaming others or enacting cruelty on others?*

8 **Are they able to forgive or let go of disappointments, or once you hurt them, the relationship is severed?** *How might this client handle the shame and pain triggered in a relationship when someone hurts them in connection with their marginalized status? Do they sever the relationship after one microaggression? Or do they work it through if the person is willing?*

9 **Do they react differently when someone disappoints them vs. being disappointed in themselves?**

10 **How do they respond to feedback from others when a person expresses disappointment in them or delivers constructive criticism which is meant to be helpful?**

In the initial assessment phase of treatment, we can begin to appreciate how adding questions that reflect a cultural perspective provides a richer understanding regarding the impact that privilege and/or marginalization can have on one's sense of identity. The level of specificity of these questions is aimed at opening a doorway of communication, one that conveys respect for the client's heritage, socioeconomic status, and uniqueness. Most clients who do not hold a position of privilege in our culture are hesitant to reveal the hidden parts of themselves, fearing that they will be misunderstood or minimized. These questions convey that the therapist is aware of dynamics around micro-aggression and how these less than fully conscious assumptions contribute to and reinforce a sense of marginalization.

Much of the content material that *all* clients initially bring into therapy represents only a partial view of the etiology of their pain and suffering. Over time, however, careful inquiry will help to reveal more of a complete picture. Throughout the treatment process, as we continue to see further dimensions of the psyche, we begin to understand the value of psychodynamic formulation in terms of how it can be used as a barometer of the evolving therapeutic process over time. Drawing upon the language and concepts illustrated in the Healthy Self-Actualizing Model can also assist in penetrating defensively based beliefs by posing alternative ways of approaching life that are more balanced and integrated.

Psychodynamic Formulation Template Using the Four Quadrant Model

Below you will find a sample grid that organizes a case formulation into component parts. Not all parts may be known during the initial assessment phase, but they can be filled in as more relevant case information is revealed throughout the course of treatment. Depending on your theoretical orientation, you may elect to eliminate sections within this template and add relevant sections of your own.

This template is divided into four sections – *Identifying Information, Part-Whole Analysis, Quality of Navigating/Functioning in the World,* and *Predictive Projections* in terms of treatment outcome. Each of the sections have bulleted items and/or questions attached to help you complete the formulation. Not all of the bulleted items under each question will apply to each individual case. The art of writing a succinct formulation is to capture the most relevant aspects of the case which will be highlighted within the case formulation write-up.

The detail that is covered in this template is meant to help you think about the most relevant aspects of each case. For example, if your client is a Caucasian, middle class, cis-gender, straight female, the section on Cultural Factors may or may not be as relevant as how you might think about the case if your client is a first generation American or a person of color. If your patient has a trauma history, the section on developmental history, their learned "loyalty contracts," and how they navigate the world may be of particular significance. Individuals with early attachment/regulation deficits and other forms of complex trauma experience life through a brain that is wired differently than individuals who developed in a secure environment. Without going into detail, it is sufficient to say that the more primitive areas of the brain, the brain stem and limbic system, are more active in the networks of the brain of traumatized individuals, and the prefrontal cortex is less hardwired into the networks. This results in more fear, hypervigilance, and negative rumination. Paying attention to the degree that vigilance and safety concerns influence how decisions are made will be useful. This includes attending to the degree to which a client misinterprets cues in the environment both interpersonal and institutional. It is important to remember that all the questions identified in the bulleted sections do not need to be answered to complete a thorough psychodynamic formulation.

Psychodynamic Formulation Template

Part One: Identifying Information

- Presenting Concern & Precipitating Event (What brings patient to therapy)
- Demographic Information – age, marital status, race, gender identity, country of origin, sexual orientation, disability status, class/economic advantage or disadvantage, primary language, religion, education
- Mood, demeanor, physical presentation
- Medical or health concerns if relevant
- Prior therapy, quality of attachment to prior therapist, length of time in treatment.

Part Two: Part-Whole Analysis

1   ATTACHMENT HISTORY – **(Quadrant One and Three)** Describe the patient's relevant developmental history in terms of:

- Secure, Insecure Ambivalent, Insecure Avoidant, Disorganized
- Were there relevant events within the family system that impacted security, safety, opportunity?
- Connect early attachment history to the degree of trauma, abuse, deprivation
- Were there any positive attachment figures outside of family of origin?

2   CHARACTER SOLUTION – **(Quadrant One)** Describe your initial impression of the patient's overdetermined beliefs, behaviors, using the three Character Solutions – Moving Toward, Moving Away, Moving Against)

- Assess the degree of rigidity or compulsivity of the defensive construction.
- What is the level of shame sensitivity that underlies the Character Solution?
- How does the defensive "solution" appear to tax the individual and/or the individual's relationships? (**Symptom breakthrough Quadrant Two**)
- How does the person feel about needing/receiving help?

3   CORE CONFLICT/LOYALTY CONTRACT – **(Quadrant Three)** Describe the patient's conflict around the unspoken or spoken loyalty contract requiring self-sacrifice in order to maintain safety and connection.

- Describe any fears the patient harbors if the loyalty contract is broken.
- Describe any harbored resentments if the loyalty contract is kept.
- How much of the authentic self has had to be sacrificed in order to preserve the tenuous attachment bond created by the loyalty contract?

4   REPEATED PATTERNS – **(Quadrant Three and Four)** How does the core conflict or learned loyalty contract manifest through "enactments" in current relationships?

- What are their hidden fears, wishes, and/or longings for rescue?
- How does the patient handle disappointment?
- What is the degree of fairness/sense of mutuality the client brings to relationships?
- What are shame triggers, and what attempts does the patient use to hide feelings of shame or inadequacy?

5   CULTURAL FACTORS – That Impact Symptoms, Self-Worth, Agency, Opportunity (**Quadrant One**)

- What is the client's race, ethnicity, immigration status?
- What degree of cultural marginalization has the client incorporated into narrative?
- Is your client a first, second, third generation American citizen, and how might this play out in terms of identity, individuation, and loyalty?
- Are there cultural beliefs, taboos that may challenge the therapeutic process?

Part Three: Quality of Navigating/Functioning in the World

1   CAPACITIES AROUND DECISION-MAKING PROCESSES (**Quadrant One**)

- **Intentionality**

- Are decisions made with forethought and sense of purpose?
- Are decisions fraught with unrealistic fears and apprehensions?
- Is there an impulsive quality to decision-making, i.e., living for the moment or being swept away by emotion?
- Is there an overly cautious/ruminative quality to decision-making?

- **Passive resignation**

  - Does personal initiative trigger fears of reprisal, personal threat or negative consequences?
  - Is there an overall sense of passivity, waiting for others to provide answers?
  - Is there a feeling of hopelessness with regard to initiating or completing tasks?

- **Commitment conflict**

  - Is commitment perceived as an entrapment or opportunity?
  - How does the patient understand/describe avoidance of commitment?

- **Spontaneity**

  - What is the level of rigidity in decision making and daily routine?
  - How easy is it for the individual to change plans, accommodate disruptions in routine?

- **Curiosity**

  - How easy is it for the individual to take in new information and adapt beliefs and assumptions accordingly?
  - What is the level of self-reflective capacity?

2 STRENGTHS, RESOURCES, SOCIAL SUPPORTS **(Healthy Self Model)**

- What is the quality of friendships – number of friends, longevity of friendships?
- What social interests/hobbies/creative outlets does the patient have?
- What level of financial security/insecurity does the patient have?
- Describe the patient's relationship to extended family.
- How satisfying is the patient's occupation/employment situation?

3 CAPACITIES THAT MEASURE AFFECT REGULATION – What is the degree of self-regulation, affective awareness, reactivity? **(Quadrant Two & Four)**

- **How frequently does the individual lose his/her temper?**

- Is the memory that triggers affective arousal clearly know or is it unformulated?
- How does the person justify or explain temper outburst?
- Is there any shame attached to these episodes?

- **How much does negative self-criticism interfere with moving forward in life?**

  - Do their ruminations around perfectionism interfere with completing simple task?
  - How much time are they spending ruminating on events?
  - What is their capacity to self-soothe or stop anxiety and ruminative focus on the self?
  - What is their degree of hypervigilance?
  - How much awareness do they have in terms of understanding the role self-criticism plays in self-regulation?
  - Do they connect their self-critical voice with parental messages around achievement and self-worth?

- **Do they use any other motivators other than criticism to try accomplish tasks?**
- **What self-regulation attempts do they use to cope?**

  - Addictions - Alcohol and substances, Food, Gaming, Exercise, Pornography
  - Withdrawal from interpersonal contact

- **How do they resolve conflicts or disappointments that trigger shame?**

  - Complete cutting off of the person
  - Retaliation
  - Talking it through
  - Forgiveness and letting go

Part Four: Predictive Projections/ Treatment Plan:

1   What are the patient's internal strengths "ego capacities" and/or motivations that may predict outcome success of treatment?
2   How might the patient's patterns or enactments eventually play out in the treatment relationship? (What do you anticipate in terms of transferential and potential counter-transferential reactions?)
3   Does the patient have suitable resources and support networks that would allow for long-term psychotherapy?
4   What form of therapy will best suit this client given the above factors?

Example of a Case Formulation Write-Up Using the Four Quadrant Template

A case sample is provided below. It is aimed at providing an illustration of how the psychodynamic case formulation template can be used in setting treatment goals, as well as acting as a dynamic snapshot of the client at any given moment of time during the treatment.

Part One: Identifying Information

Maya is a bi-racial, 34-year-old, cisgender female who is recently divorced from her husband whom she met while travelling in Mexico at the age of 26. Husband came to the US with the plan to marry so that he could claim US citizenship. They have one daughter, age four. Precipitating events that brought this patient into therapy center around the divorce and a custody battle over their daughter. Patient's concern over shared custody is that husband has had a history of verbal abuse and appears to be minimally attached to daughter. Husband has had a spotty work history throughout their relationship, and Maya often had to work over-time to make ends meet. When she tried to confront her husband about finding a job or taking over some of the responsibility for their daughter, he became cold and distant, saying she didn't appreciate him enough. At that point, her husband began having an affair which eventually led to their divorce. Maya states that she doesn't trust her husband and reports that he has threatened to take their daughter to Mexico if he does not receive joint custody rights.

This is the first time the patient has entered therapy and presents with symptomatic complaints of depression, lethargy, and anxiety with epi-sodic panic attacks. Patient presents as well-groomed, educated, and articulate. She is employed as a paralegal in a top law firm in the city. There are no relevant health concerns, however, there is a family history of depression and anxiety on maternal side of family. On initial contact, Maya presented with a shy demeanor, anxiety, tearfulness, and had difficulty expressing what she wanted from therapy. She did become somewhat more relaxed as the session continued and reported that she felt relief telling her story.

Part Two: Part-Whole Analysis

Patient's family history reveals a relatively insecure parental attachment due to mother's chronic episodes of depression and lack of availability. Maya's mother, a Caucasian, married a Hispanic man when they were both in their late teens. Parental relationship was filled with episodic fighting, where father would storm out of the house, leaving mother and three children alone for days at a time. When Maya was eight years of age, mother asked her husband to leave for reasons that remain unclear. After the divorce, father returned to Mexico, never to be seen again. Maya is angry and confused about this and blames father for leaving mother with such a difficult life. After the divorce Maya's mother had to work full-time, and she remembers her mother being tearful and exhausted most of the time. One particularly fond memory Maya does have is that she would make breakfast for her mother on Saturday mornings. Mother would let her come up into bed and snuggle, and she would tell Maya how much she appreciated her helping with her younger siblings. Her mother told her that God rewards people for their sacrifice, just like mom has had to sacrifice for their family. This left an indelible impression on Maya, who states that her aim in life is to make people happy.

As an adult Maya actively seeks out relationships and tries to be a helpful and loving to her friends and family. As the oldest of three siblings, Maya's caretaking role in adulthood extends to partially supporting her brother's children financially, even though her brother has failed to repay past loans on numerous occasions. Maya's character solution appears to be Moving Toward, putting other's needs ahead of her own. She experiences spikes in anxiety if she feels she has fallen short of friends or family members' expectations. It is unclear at this point the degree of shame sensitivity that drives the character solution, but Maya does admit she is not as smart as other co-workers in her legal firm, and spends hours taking work home in order to meet her boss's expectations and high standards.

These over-determined efforts at work and with family take a toll on Maya as she chronically reports getting little sleep many work nights. She suffers from fatigue, often skips lunch, and feels guilty for not being able to spend enough time with her daughter. The degree of anxiety around perceived shortcomings in any area of her life can at times trigger panic attacks. This is especially true around work deadlines or when she ruminates about her husband kidnapping their daughter and taking her to Mexico. Maya admits having difficulty receiving help from others; however, she does seem amenable to utilizing therapy and has been gradually able to reveal more about her fears of being alone or having her daughter taken from her.

The patient's core relational conflict can be articulated as a loyalty issue that is connected to her mother's suffering and Maya's belief that if she gives enough of herself, she can relieve other people's burdens, that relationships will stay intact and people won't leave her. The loyalty contract can be articulated in quid pro quo terms as – *If I give all of myself to you, I will be able to help you enough so that you will see my value and appreciate me, and then you will take care of me and won't leave me like my father did. If I try to stand up for myself and ask for my needs to be met, I will fall short in God's eyes, it will only burden people and they will get angry, and eventually leave me.*

Within session Maya often expresses confusion around whether she has a right to ask for her own needs to be met. She seems to have a great deal of confusion differentiating between self-care and selfishness. Her resentments around maintaining the loyalty contract are directed toward others in that she doesn't think it's fair that other people get away with being irresponsible when she works so hard to do the right thing. She does harbor some resentment that the world is unfair but tries to comfort herself by taking the position that God will provide. Essentially, she has adopted more a resigned position and appears to be unaware as to the cost this is taking. She does not seem to have a clear sense of what constitutes fairness and mutuality in a relationship and ends up repeatedly getting disappointed or taken advantage of by co-workers and family members. Maya appears to "loyally wait" for someone to recognize her efforts so that she can receive reward and praise. When praise is not forthcoming, Maya turns this disappointment against herself, saying she could have done more.

Cultural factors that may have an impact on Maya's sense of self-worth are that she is afraid of being seen as a "mixed breed." She seems to have internalized a negative introject about being less-than because she is not fully white and not fully Hispanic. She states that she doesn't feel that she really belongs anywhere and feels like an outcast, citing evidence that many of the white girls in the office never ask her to meet for a drink after work. To compensate for her sense of isolation, she works to prove her worth by accomplishing more than others at work, hoping for recognition and advancement to prove herself.

Part Three: Quality of Navigating/Functioning in the World

Maya is highly intentional and driven when it comes to achieving her goals. However, this intentionality and focus in her efforts seems to be over-determined as measured by her inability to take breaks, her lack of self-care, and her unawareness that overwork is affecting symptom break-through. Furthermore, she exhibits signs of passive resignation in terms of being able to change her disenfranchised status in the workplace. Although she has a curiosity about learning and taking on new projects, again they seem to be in the service of keeping anxiety and insecurity at bay. Much of her effort seems to be dedicated to safety and security, and there is little evidence that she has much time for outside interests, creative endeavors, or spontaneity. Life seems to be lived on a survival-level mode.

This is further confirmed by examining the quality of Maya's self-regulatory capacities and her own affective self-awareness. She exhibits a great deal of negative self-criticism and self-doubt that seems to be interfering with her efficiency in performing tasks. She reports ruminations around whether she completed a work assignment well enough, with hopes of achieving near perfectionistic standards. This leaves her exhausted with little ability to stop the ruminations or use self-soothing capacities to rest and restore. However, Maya has not exhibited any addictive behaviors to relieve stress and/or calm ruminative thoughts. She reports that playing with her daughter and reading to her in the evenings helps to calm her down.

An initial goal of treatment would be to focus on increasing Maya's external support systems in an effort to help create life-style balance and relieve day-to-day stress. She does have several close friends from childhood that she calls upon which provide her a sense of comfort and continuity. However, friends in her current community environment seem to be lacking. Encouraging her to pursue a social activity or creative pursuit on the weekends might decrease stress and social isolation. Family and work are her top priorities, and Maya seems to take a great deal of pride and satisfaction out of work, despite the stress it causes her. In spite of Maya's current external stress and ruminative anxiety around the divorce and custody battle, she does seem to exhibit signs of resilience when it comes to caring for her daughter, saying she will not give up and she will use her "resources and her wits" to make sure her daughter is kept safe and not taken from her.

Part Four: Predictive Projections / Treatment Plan

Maya has shown increased motivation to continue with the therapy process after the initial assessment process. She has already experienced a good deal of symptom relief by simply being able to talk about her ruminations and her fears around the custody battle. As a result, her sleep patterns and mood seem to be improving. Given her history around motivation to finish her college degree, being the first member of her family to do so, Maya shows the strength and resilience to engage in long-term psychotherapy. Maya has a solid work ethic and is able to bring her curiosity, creativity, and analytic abilities to her work efforts. That energy could be harnessed and channeled toward in-depth psychotherapy if she continues to show interest and motivation to do so.

The patient's patterns around attachment injury and her longings for caretaking/recognition by a nurturing authority figure may initially play out by developing an idealizing transference with a need to overly please the therapist. It would be important for the therapist to look for opportunities to invite Maya to show all aspects of herself, especially where there may be areas of harbored resentment or disappointment. Since there was a family taboo around expressing negative feelings, the patient may initially hide these aspects of herself from the therapeutic dialogue. Possible negative transferential feelings toward her therapist who is a Caucasian female may play out around trust issues about her internalized feelings around feeling marginalized and therefore possibly misunderstood.

The patient has resources through her company's insurance policy to be able to make a commitment to long-term therapy. The most suitable form of therapy for this patient would be a combination of a cognitive-behavioral approach using systematic desensitization for anxiety and ruminations coupled with a psychodynamic approach to focus on relational patterns, feelings of poor self-worth and developing a more secure attachment pattern. The aim of longer-term work would be to help Maya adjust her expectations around what constitutes fairness and mutuality in relationships and how to directly advocate for herself without over-compensating in an attempt to prove her worthiness.

Chapter Summary

The aim of a psychodynamic case formulation is to create a snapshot of the human psyche at any given point in time. And as good photographer knows, creating a good snapshot requires knowledge of depth of field, adjusting the camera settings in a way that the lens is able to capture the right elements of both figure and ground.

The therapeutic stance needed to capture both figure and ground of our clients' full humanity is at heart of what constitutes a rich and meaningful psychodynamic formulation. The ability to see more of the subtle nuances of the complexity of the psyche as well as the changing theoretical field and ground of case conceptualization increases as one's therapeutic stance matures. Continually revisiting a client's case formulation throughout the treatment process is an invitation to let go of assumptions and reassess with fresh eyes. In the most basic sense, the invitation is toward listening with deeper curiosity, stretching us to hear what our clients are trying to say, both through their verbal articulations as well as through non-verbal enactments.

Clinical observation and scientific research are providing us with a more detailed roadmap in terms of confirming and expanding the numerous factors that are necessary to complete a thorough assessment and effective treatment plan. When we sit down to write a case formulation, we are reminded of the importance of challenging ourselves to think about what we might not be seeing, to continually wonder how our own training methods as well as our internalized blind spots and biases may limit us. As the field moves toward further dimensions of therapeutic integration, we have become more aware of the impact that trauma, deprivation, privilege, race, and class have had on shaping our theoretical assumptions. With each expansion of theoretical understanding, we are able to incorporate these important discoveries into the nature of the human suffering and resilience. The elements and measures included in this chapter hopefully will add additional ways of holding both the macro and micro view of dynamic formulation.

References

Akhtar, S. (1992). *Understanding human nature.* Garden City Publishing.

Benjamin, L. S. (1993). *Interpersonal diagnosis and treatment of personality disorders.* Guilford Press.

Bucci, W. (2011). The role of embodied communication in therapeutic change: A multiple code perspective. In W. Tschacher & C. Bergomi, (Eds.), *The Role of embodied communication in therapeutic change.* (pp. 209–228). Imprint Academic.

Elliott, R., Greenberg, L. S., & Lietaer, G. (2004). Research on experiential psychotherapies. In M. J. Lambert (Ed.), *Bergein & Garfield's handbook of psychotherapy and behavior change* (5th ed., pp. 493–539). Wiley.

Friedman, R. S., & Lister, P. (1987). The current status of psychodynamic formulation. *Psychiatry, 50,* 126–141.

Greenberg, L. S., Rice, L. N., & Elliott, R. (1993). *Facilitating emotional change: The moment-by-moment process.* Guilford Press.

Goldman, R. N. & Greenberg, L. S. (2015). *Case formulation in emotion-focused therapy: Co-creating clinical maps for change.* American Psychological Association.

Johnson, S. M. (1994). *Character styles.* Norton.

Josephs, L. (1992). *Character structure and the organization of the self.* Columbia University Press.

Kernberg, O. (1984). *Severe personality disorders: Psychotherapeutic strategies.* Yale University Press.

Lyons-Ruth, K., Dutra, L., Schuder, M., & Banchi, L. (2006). From infant attachment disorganization to adult dissociation: Relational adaptations for traumatic experiences. *Psychiatric Clinics of North America, 29*(1), 63–86.

MacKinnon, R. A., & Michels, R. (1971). *The psychiatric interview in clinical practice.* Saunders.

McWilliams, N. (1999). *Psychoanalytic case formulation.* Guilford Press.

Millon, T. (1981). *Disorder of Personality: DMS- III: Axis II.* Wiley.

Othmer, E., & Othmer, S. C. (1989). *The clinical interview: Using DSM-III-R.* American Psychiatric Press.

Orange, D. M., Atwood, G. E., & Stolorow, R. D. (1997). *Working intersubjectively: Contextualism in psychoanalytic practice.* Routledge.

Perry S., Cooper, A. M., & Michels, R. (1987). The psychodynamic formulation: It's purpose, structure, and clinical application. *American Journal of Psychiatry, 144*(5), 543–550.

Rice, L. N., & Greenberg, L. S. (Eds.). (1984). *Patterns of change: An intensive analysis of psychotherapeutic process.* Guilford Press.

Schore, J. R., & Schore, A. N. (2008). Modern attachment theory: The central role of affect regulation in development and treatment. *Clinical Social Work Journal, 36.*

Stolorow, R. D. (2013). Intersubjective-systems theory: A phenomenological-contextualist psychoanalytic perspective. *Psychoanalytic Dialogues, 23,* 383–389. Routledge: Taylor Francis Group.

Stolorow, R. D., Brandchaft, B., & Atwood, G. E. (1987). *Psychoanalytic treatment: An intersubjective approach.* The Analytic Press.

Summers, R. F. (2003). The psychodynamic formulation updated. *American Journal of Psychotherapy, 57*(1), 39–51.

Wachtel, P. L. (2014). *Cyclical psychodynamics and the contextual self: The inner world, the intimate world, and the world of culture and society.* Routledge.

4 Getting Beneath the Tip of the Iceberg: How to Use Entry Points in Language to Uncover Hidden Material

Introduction

Language is important. It is, after all, the major tool we rely on in "talk therapy." Yet, talk therapy has many divergent branches, and each theoretical approach varies greatly in terms of *how therapists listen* to what they hear and *how they derive meaning* from what is conveyed. Our theoretical orientation influences both what draws our clinical attention and also what escapes our view. This chapter is aimed at presenting a way of listening and tracking that can be replicated across multiple theoretical disciplines, one that may hopefully create a more unifying standard in terms of how to delve more deeply into the dialogic exchange between patient and therapist.

As Donnel Stern (2015) states, "Language is not only a medium for the representation of meaning that already exists; it also actually participates in the creation of meaning. The nature of our thoughts or experiences – whatever one wants to call the products of the activities of the mind – are deeply influenced by language" (p. 87). Focusing on the patient's language and affective resonance in the unfolding present allows us to stay *with* the patient. Slowing down the dialogic process and listening for what is about to emerge in the moment contributes greatly to the creation of a therapeutic holding environment. This quality of attention, where our patients can be witnessed, understood, and encouraged, is what eventually allows for the letting go of limiting beliefs and behaviors.

The first technique to be introduced in this text provides a way for therapists to listen to the client's use of language as a means of gaining further insight into material that is known, partially know, or outside of the client's awareness altogether. Tracking "entry points" in the communication is a method that illustrates how to catch more of the story, hold more of the suffering, cut through more of the isolation, so that what is hidden, unacknowledged, or unformulated can be revealed and held in the present moment. This method of tracking is also what helps to minimize the risk of moving too quickly into our assumptions rather than letting the client's process show us where to direct our attention. Attending to the rhythm of

DOI: 10.4324/9781003120278-5

language, and to non-verbal cues moment-to-moment is how the conveyance of shared meaning is articulated through the verbal exchange.

Often our patients will say a word or a phrase, and they will assume you understand what they mean, even though very little specific information may have been given. For the person who is receiving the information, it's almost as if they are listening to someone who is speaking in code. For example, a patient may say, *"My mother was a saint,"* and will expect you to know what that means. You may hear this as a simple, seemingly straightforward statement; yet, under the surface we get the sense that there is likely to be a great deal of hidden information.

As a therapist you may be thinking... *What mother is really a saint? What might my patient be trying to convey to me about his family of origin? Was he given no choice other than to believe his mother was a saint? What might that say about his mother's relational expectations, her fragility, or her rage? Does the patient have other emotions about his mother that may run counter to this belief about her sainthood? Are those emotions too threatening to acknowledge consciously? How did that dynamic come into being?*

Uncovering the answers to these questions is not always an easy, straightforward task. Certainly, how we enter into the inquiry process must always begin in a way that is delicate enough so as not to overwhelm the client. Timing and level of trust are key factors when considering any type of clinical intervention. Furthermore, we must be mindful to guard against our own assumptions coloring or clouding the direction of the inquiry. How do we allow what might be under the surface to emerge in a way that is neutral enough, but curious enough so that we can more accurately see where the client's process will lead?

Within any given therapeutic exchange, a client's verbal communication is often more complex than the surface conversation may imply. Clients will reveal certain parts of their narrative, while other parts are consciously withheld, or they are underneath conscious awareness all together. Too often words and phrases that potentially convey hidden meaning slip right by because we haven't developed a keen enough listening ear to catch a phrase that may telegraph that there is more to the story. For example, therapists, who over-attend to the content of what a patient is saying, or therapists who push to find solutions to a patient's complaints often miss critical opportunities that could have afforded them a window into richer, more tender aspects of the patient's inner world.

Paying attention to what is being conveyed in between the lines of the communication is precisely how we begin to attend to process dynamics. This quality of attention not only helps us learn more about our clients' beliefs or values, it also allows us to observe the quality of their thinking, the level of depth and curiosity they have about the world, how open or closed they are to new ideas, and how much of their reactions are triggered by perceived emotional slights. It also lets us see how frequently they use language to over-compensate in order to present a positive self-image, or how much of what they express is aimed at pleasing others. This way of listening to language as an entry point into deeper exploration, is the focus of this chapter.

How to Spot an Entry Point

In our second book, *Uncovering the Resilient Core,* Jack Danielian and I define an entry point as a way therapists can use the patient's language as a tracking process to learn more about:

- How patients think and organize information.
- What they perceive and what they fail to perceive.
- The affective meaning of a given event.
- The level of intensity of frustrations and disappointments.
- The speed of their reactivity to a situation.
- The underlying assumptions and hidden expectations of self and others.
- How the perceived self-system is organized.

Generally, where there was a history of early attachment failure, either through trauma, deprivation, or narcissistic enmeshment, individuals carry an internal sense of inadequacy buried at the core of "who I am." These children grow into adulthood feeling ill-equipped to move through the world with ease, or they secretly feel like a fraud even in the face of success. How they communicate and organize their thinking is in part used to hide feelings of unworthiness both from self and from others.

Early in treatment when entering into dialogue, you may find that these patients display a tendency to overly please the therapist by being a good patient, or you will find a patient who displays more rigidity in thinking, coupled with a refusal to challenge one's own assumptions, as if there is an "impenetrability" to their organizing schema. Establishing trust takes much time, and the patient's demands of proof that test the therapeutic relationship are part of the journey. Here is where the therapist must tread carefully when using language as an entry point into deeper inquiry. Here is also where repetition, coming back to material again and again, becomes part of the nuance of using this technique.

Listening for language that may be an entry point into deeper material can seem somewhat of a subjective experience at first. With practice, however, words or phrases that contain hidden meaning become easier to identify. By paying attention to the patient's tone of voice, attending to when there is avoidance of eye contact, or when you notice subtle shifts in body language can also be non-verbal cues that help the therapist spot material which telegraphs that there is something further to be explored. By slowing down the process and asking for further clarification, a fuller picture often emerges.

For example, if a patient declares, *"I'm just fine. I pride myself in being able to keep my emotions under control,"* the therapist's task is to then try to get beneath the surface of this statement. What does "just fine" mean? Why is pride associated with not showing emotions? The therapist's next statement would be key to opening up the entry point to gain further understanding. There are numerous choices as to how the therapist might respond, and there is never only one right response. Here are just a few examples of what a therapist might say next.

- *When you say you're just fine, I'm wondering, what does that mean to you?*
- *When you keep your emotions under control, you feel a sense of pride? Tell me more about how that might make you feel good about yourself?*
- *You told me that you're fine, but what you were sharing seemed to be very sad and painful. Can you tell me how you are able to make yourself feel just fine?*
- *You just said that you take pride in keeping your emotions under control. I'm curious. As a child, what did you observe about how your parents expressed their emotions?*
- *I noticed that you started to tear up, and then you pulled yourself together and said you're just fine. What just happened in that moment?*

The list of examples can go on and on. The point is that the therapist's task is to take a significant part of the patient's actual statement and reflect those words back to the patient, then ask for further clarification. Additionally, the therapist's task is to notice what happened moments before the entry point declaration was made. In this way the therapist may be able to articulate a connection between unconscious or split off material to statements, beliefs, or assumptions that are consciously understood by the patient. It also conveys that we are giving our patients our undivided attention, noticing the verbal and non-verbal cues within any given exchange.

Tracking inconsistencies in the thread of the conversation is another way to use language as a means of discovering parts of the patient's narrative that are split off from the larger whole. For example, does the content of what a patient is telling us completely contradict what he or she had said previously? Does the verbal content match what we are picking up affectively or non-verbally, right-brain-to-right brain? Does the patient shift away from material too quickly when asked for clarification? Often, we may sense an undercurrent of a feeling, even though a feeling is being denied, or we may sense a feeling of discomfort and are not sure where it is coming from.

Here are several examples that illustrate where more clarification is required to obtain a fuller picture of what the patient means.

I feel like I've turned a corner with my boyfriend Steve.
You'll probably disagree with me when I say this, but...

I feel like I have to walk on eggshells.
Well, you know what it's been like for me.
Don't you agree that most people end up disappointing you sooner or later?
I'm a pretty open book. I say what's on my mind and don't hold back.
It's been a pretty rough week.
I'm sick and tired of people who don't pull their own weight.
You and I both know that my wife tends to over-react?
You're the only person that I feel won't disappoint me.
Not much has been happening. I have nothing much to report.

As you can see each of these phrases convey a piece of information, but the full meaning remains unclear. Accessing the detail requires developing the art of knowing what to say next. A simple way to begin entry point tracking is to simply repeat the patient's statement or choose a part of the statement, using the exact wording to ask for further clarification.

For example, if a patient says, "You and I both know that my wife tends to over-react," you may focus on the word *over-react* and ask, "What do you mean, over-react" or "Can you give me an example of what she did that felt like an over-reaction?" On the other hand, you may choose to comment on what the patient might be assuming when he says, *you and I both know,* and repeat his opening phrase by putting the phrase back to the patient in the form of a question, stating, "You and I both know?"

What comes next is the beginning of a tracking process where you follow the dialogic exchange as it unfolds. The patient's next statement will generally give you a little more information that then leads you to the next entry point, allowing you to go a little deeper into the patient's feelings or assumptions.

Here might be one way that this conversation might play out a little further. The potential words that are entry points are underlined. Notice that when using the technique of working with an entry point phrase and asking for more detail, it will often lead to a statement where the patient reveals another entry point in need of clarification.

Pt: *"You and I both know that my wife tends to over-react."*
Th: *"What do you mean, over-react?"*
Pt: *"Well you know, I've talked about this before."*
Th: *"Could you give me an example of something that happened this week where she over-reacted?"*
Pt: *"She got upset because I forgot to take out the trash, but I had a really hectic week, and I was out of town and came in late. I don't know why she couldn't be more understanding."*
Th: *So, you were hoping she'd be more understanding? What did that feel like when she wasn't?"*
Pt: *"Like I said, I shouldn't be surprised. She always over-reacts. I guess all women are a little too emotional."*

Th: *"So, you handled your disappointment with your wife by telling yourself that all women are a little too emotional? Don't you have a right to feel disappointed?"*

Pt: *"I know I shouldn't lump all women into the same category. You're right, I was disappointed, and I was a little angry if you must know. Sometimes it makes me feel hopeless that she'll ever really be there for me."*

Th: *"And that feeling of hopelessness makes you tell yourself that all women are too emotional. Does that make you feel less angry with your wife?"*

Pt: *"Yes, it's what makes me keep hanging in there. I guess I tell myself, what's the point in making a fuss. All women are just so sensitive. It's easier to keep my mouth shut."*

Th: *"How is that easier?"*

Clearly this conversation could have also gone in several different directions. Let's say in this instance the patient's therapist was a woman. What may be being telegraphed is something that is transferential in nature, and the inquiry process could have gone in that direction just as easily. We will use this same client example in Chapter Seven on working with transferential communication to illustrate how to use entry point communication to draw out latent transferential material.

Holding Multiple Parts Simultaneously: Connecting Entry Points to the Four Quadrant Model

In the early phase of therapeutic inquiry, one of our tasks is to identify repeated patterns in our patients' communication style. We make note of what our clients pay attention to and what triggers an emotional reaction of hyper-reactivity or shutdown. We also notice what is minimized, areas of the psyche that seem to be under-reported or hidden from view. Here is where applying the Four Quadrant Model to our patients' communication style can be quite useful. By listening for which quadrants occupy the patient's psychic attention, as well as which quadrants seem under-developed or under-represented, a picture begins to emerge where we can then recognize how a patient's over-determined efforts work to keep intense feelings that threaten to overwhelm psychic equilibrium from coming to the surface. For example, the amount of time a client focuses energy on efforts to succeed and reach perfectionistic standards (Q1) at the expense of life style balance (Q2) is a coping strategy that is not sustainable over time. When we are able to tune ourselves to these balances and imbalances, we can more clearly understand how a patient's thoughts, feelings, and behaviors may also be attempts to hide or compensate for feelings of shame or inadequacy.

When we spot a phrase that may be an entry point, we are trying to access feelings that may be too painful for the individual to acknowledge consciously or to expose in the presence of another. In doing so, we gradually begin to cut through feelings of isolation, confusion, and alone-ness. We then encourage patients to elaborate on thoughts that are not clearly formulated or are based on assumptions that may not be accurate. We are also looking for the link between affective memory triggers and what the patient reflexively does in response to being triggered. In turn we try to normalize uncomfortable feelings and give reassurance in an effort to minimize feelings of shame. In sum working with language as an entry point creates a safe holding environment for hidden material to eventually surface.

Once we are able to get beneath the surface dialogue, we are able to uncover fractures or hidden parts of the personality. As we continue to follow the dialogic exchange, we listen and wait for where those hidden parts of the self will lead us. It's much like pulling on a thread in a sweater and seeing how it begins to unravel. As we pull on the language thread, we discover that with more careful inquiry, the defenses gradually begin to unravel on their own, revealing more tender parts that have been lying in waiting. If we create a safe enough holding environment, and we attune ourselves carefully and skillfully enough, we discover that the authentic self has its own energy and desire to emerge. Parts of the self that had to be disavowed are able to be integrated into an ever-expanding whole.

It is our job to hold the various parts of the psyche simultaneously, even when the patient cannot. This is where the Four Quadrant Model can assist as a road map in terms of informing us where to look and what to ask. For example, a patient may present a pattern where devaluing of others oc-cupies much of the dialogue, where much of the patient's energy and focus is on Quadrant Four. Anger is the prevailing affect expressed in each session due to repeated experiences of disappointment. However, upon closer inspection, the patient's expectations of self are also over-determined/perfectionistic. There is little if any access to feelings of vulnerability. In the following client example, the therapist recognized potential underlying themes within the devaluing phrases. She then began to explore which quadrants were at play in terms of understanding more the patient's re-peated defense pattern more fully.

Client Example

This is a young woman who came from a divorced family and lived with a mother who was very cold and critical. Nothing that the daughter did was ever good enough. Mother was self-centered, demanding, and emotionally labile. If the daughter dared to ask for mother's help or if she showed any display of emotion, she was told that she was weak, disgusting, and the mother wished she had never been born. The therapist admitted that working with this client was rather difficult because the therapist couldn't find any way to penetrate the client's angry defense. In an attempt to connect the patient's defensively based entry point language to the Four

Quadrant Model, the therapist provided a list of phrases that her client tended to repeat in almost every session. The words that are underlined draw our attention to the client's devaluing of others and are entry points into further exploration.

I'm just trying to stay alive, but people are assholes.
People are out to screw you, but I don't want to be a victim.
People can't admit that they're not good people.
There are no more options for me, and doctors are so stupid.
I do everything right, and I never feel better.
There are a lot of people who feel sorry for themselves, but I don't.

You can see how the patient uses anger and devaluing in Quadrant Four to manage her disappointment and feelings of hopelessness. However, when you study these phrases as a whole, it becomes clear that the patient's extremely high standard for herself in Quadrant One, and her equally high standard for others in Quadrant Three are what trigger the perpetual cycle of disappointment. It also telegraphs to us the patient's attempts to correct the unfair loyalty contract of her childhood by insisting on a standard of fairness that is applied equally to all.

During an initial consultation session, the therapist was asked how she handled the patient's anger and devaluing. She reported that she had tried to reflect the anger back by saying, "You sound very angry. You seem triggered." She then would ask, "What comes up for you in these moments? Why do you think you're holding onto this upset?" In each instance the client's response was to turn the dialogue away from engaging in any response that might reveal her needs, feelings of vulnerability, or any degree of self-reflection. Instead, the client would repeated turn the focus back to other people who disappointed her, giving additional details about the story and reasons why she was justified in complaining.

The therapist explained that her strategy around engaging in this approach was to try to find a way to balance or mitigate the client's anger which she experienced as intense and all-consuming. In an attempt to create a balanced perspective, the therapist would try to frame the client's disappointment and anger in a more attenuated fashion. For example, if the client called her mother a worthless jerk, the therapist would reframe this as her mother was very damaged and limited. If the client complained about her friends being selfish for not wearing masks during Covid, the therapist would try to get the client to look at it from her friends' perspective, pointing out that everyone has a right to make their own decisions. Although it might be a useful therapeutic goal to try to find ways to mitigate a client's anger, in this case the strategy of trying to calm the patient's anger wasn't working.

When anger is the prevailing and dominant emotional state in a patient, it is easy to understand how therapists might try to make attempts to help patients regulate their feelings. However, the risk in shifting away from a client's anger or disappointment too quickly often results in leaving the patient feeling misunderstood or abandoned. In this case the client may have interpreted this action as a sign that the therapist couldn't tolerate her intensity. In turn this runs the risk of activating further shame and hopelessness. Additionally, she may have perceived the therapist's comments as siding with the patient's friends or minimizing the extent of pain and damage caused by a cold and controlling mother.

At this juncture in the therapy, it was important to begin to explore what was underneath the anger and devaluing. Because this patient seemed to express her disappointment only through the devaluation of others, the therapist made the connection that the devaluing also served a function of protecting the patient from having to express her feelings of hurt or vulnerability within the therapy session. Accessing these more tender feelings would evoke too much shame around her perceived neediness. However, when the therapist tried to reflect this possibility back to the patient, the client became furious, stating that people are never held accountable for their actions, quickly pointing out that she does everything right, holds herself to a high-performance standard, doesn't feel sorry for herself, and never wants to be seen as a victim. In one consultation session, the therapist expressed her frustration stating that whatever she tried to do, the patient's frustration didn't seem to be soothed.

When a patient's strategy in Quadrant One reflects an over-determined effort to stave off feelings of helplessness, often this is a reflexive attempt at self-protection, a determination that is centered on not being taken advantage of, and not to experience feelings of sadness or self-pity. It is important to remember that this defensive response is the patient's best attempt at achieving emotional equilibrium (Q1) by giving up on the hope of ever relying on others (Q3). Conscious acknowledgement of her needs and her feelings of vulnerability must be disavowed by the patient. They are too painful to continually hold within conscious awareness. However, what is ironic is that because of this disavowal, we see the patient unconsciously adopting her mother's strategy for living – you shouldn't need anything and don't show any signs of weakness. Even though the patient had made a vow not to be like her mother in any way, she has internalized her mother's message as evidenced by the repeated enactments. Yet, her disappointment and hope for rescue remain.

A Diagrammatic Illustration of Entry Point Tracking

Using this same case, we will focus on the patient's entry point example, *"I don't want to be a victim. I don't want to feel sorry for myself"* as a means of illustrating how to use an entry point phrase to help reveal the repeated enactment. A visual illustration of an iceberg will show how the examination of the entry point phrase *"I don't want to be a victim"* can actually lead to an insight around how the patient's internalized message from mother is reenacted in the form of repeatedly devaluing others when they show any sign of weakness.

Clearly, the internalization of the enactment on the part of the patient was unconscious. The part of her that was vulnerable and needed comfort from her mother was contained consciously through the contempt she held for mother. However, treating others (and herself) as her mother had treated her was split off from conscious awareness. When the therapist pointed out the similarity, she created an opportunity for insight to help integrate part of the split off material (Figure 4.1).

Notice that when the patient continued to direct the conversation away from herself back to devaluing others, the therapist continued to address the patient's underlying vulnerability, speaking to the patient's legitimate need to be cared for by a parent. She also challenged the patient's black and white thinking around believing that people who feel sorry for themselves is the same as being selfish. By doing so, the therapist then offered an invitation to explore the possible difference between having legitimate needs and being selfish. Using entry point language in this way invites the patient to become more curious as a way of gently penetrating the mother's absolutes in terms of needs being the equivalent of neediness.

Many of us may take the phrase "I don't want to be a victim" at face value. Even though we may *think* we know what the patient means, stopping to ask for clarification can be a portal into discovering further

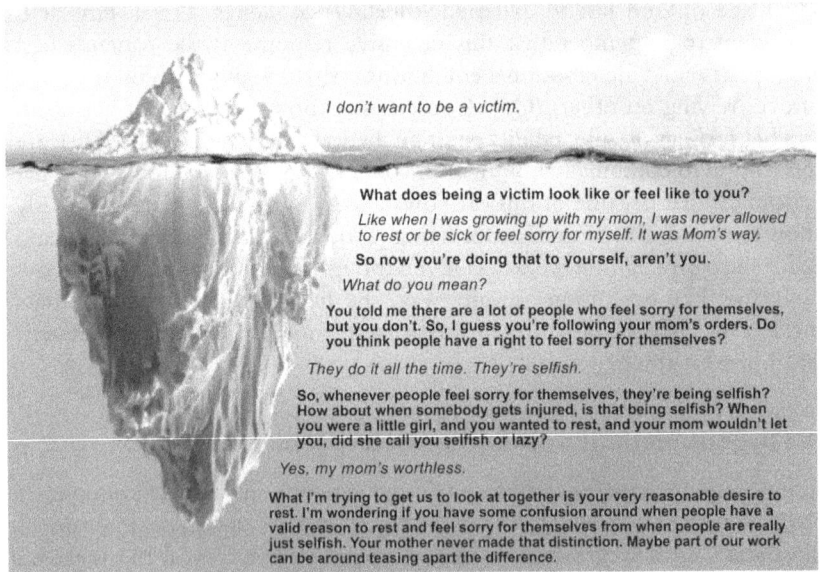

Figure 4.1 Getting Beneath the Tip of the Iceberg.

information about the patient's history as well as the patient's own assumptions about being needy or vulnerable. Although she hated her mother for not being a loving parent, the patient could not see how she had nevertheless internalized her messages through her harshness toward herself and others.

It is always a clinical judgment call as to where to direct your inquiry. In this case you could have just as easily focused on Q4, given the extent of the patient's devaluing. However, the therapist made the choice to focus on Q1 because that is where the patient's feelings of vulnerability and shame were being disavowed. Focusing on the patient's devaluing may have run the risk of evoking shame and increasing her defensiveness. Focusing on her anger runs the risk of keeping the needle in the same defensive groove. The patient needed to hear the therapist validate her right to feel vulnerable, her right to have legitimate needs that needed attention before the patient could or would be willing to adopt a gentler stance with self and eventually others.

Future work in the therapy lies in being able to use the steadiness and neutrality of the therapeutic relationship as a way to gently explore the patient's growing reliance on the therapist, which is a contrast to her experience of being with her mother. If the therapist is able to tolerate the emotional intensity of anger as the patient reveals the entry point language contained in Q4, and she is able to examine the anger more fully, *without* trying to move the patient away from her defended position, the patient hopefully will feel heard and accepted rather than being forced to move away from her right to feel and express herself. This would then allow the patient and therapist to connect present day expectations of others (Q3) with the standards she holds for herself (Q1) toward the end of adopting a less rigid, over-determined posture.

Exercise Using Entry Point Statements – Practicing What to Say Next

As a way of becoming more familiar with how to spot entry point phrases, a list of comments that patients typically make is provided below. As a practice exercise, create a list of responses that you might say next in order to gain further clarification around a potential conflict that may be hidden within the statements. You may also choose to do this exercise with a small group of colleagues. Try practicing this as a role-play exercise by engaging in a manufactured dialogue between the patient and therapist to take the exchange a bit further. For the person playing the role of the patient, give feedback to your colleague who is playing the role of the therapist in terms of how the questions and responses made you feel. Pay particular attention to aspects of the exchange that may have put you on the spot, evoking either confusion or a defensive response.

Practice Exercise – What to Say Next

"I don't know why I'm constantly disappointed by my dad."
"All I want to do is help other people. Why can't people appreciate that?"
"I don't know why I feel so angry. I know my parents were just trying to help."
"I can't be alone. I need attention to fill up the part of me that is empty."
"I can't seem to do anything right. Maybe my mother was right about me."
"I don't see what's wrong with speaking my mind. People are just too sensitive."
"I know that I'm a lot smarter than my co-workers. That's why I get impatient. I don't think I should be punished for my intelligence at work."

You will notice that each of the above statements contain some degree of hidden meaning, confusion or unresolved conflict. In addition, there is also some degree of repressed affect that is expressed within each of the statements. Several of the phases telegraph the patient's struggle around the learned loyalty contract. Others convey a pronouncement to the therapist that act almost as a subtle challenge to not disagree with their internalized beliefs and assumptions about self and other. The latter present more of a delicate challenge, as the statements reflect a transferential undercurrent that may become activated depending on how the therapist responds. Entry points in language that contain transferential cues will be covered in further detail in Chapter Seven. These entry point communications also pose a test for the therapist in terms of how to respond in a way that gathers more information while maintaining a position of neutrality.

Diagrammatic Illustration # 2 – Entry Point Tracking

In the following case we will use another diagrammatic illustration to further explore how an entry point reveals the tip of the iceberg of communication and where that leads. With this second client example we will track not only the initial conversation, but we will show how you can go back to the patient's original entry point assumption in the service of helping this patient gain mastery over a freeze response. This can be done by modeling or rehearsing a new dialogic exchange response with the client while she is not in an over-activated state. The next two diagrams include thought bubbles to help illustrate what was unspoken on the part of the patient, giving clues as to where the dialogue could lead.

No background information is needed about the case because the diagram itself will illustrate how the technique of working with entry points in language speaks for itself. The entry point phrase that the client stated upon first entering her session is *"I don't feel that I can connect to people"* (Figure 4.2).

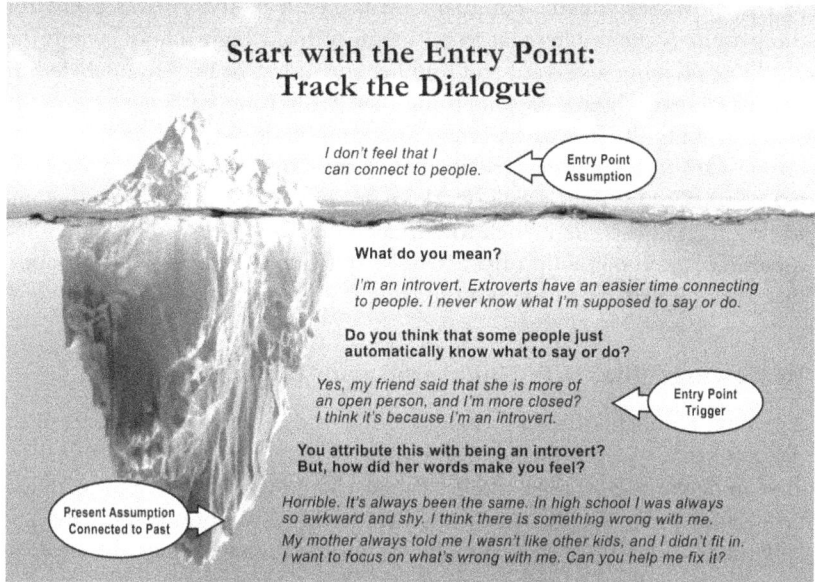

Figure 4.2 Start with the Entry Point: Track the Dialogue.

In this client example, you might be tempted to focus on the content of the patient's comment about introverts and extroverts. However, the patient's original entry point phrase spoke to a perceived shortcoming, and there is a high likelihood that feelings of disappointment or shame lie under the surface. The patient's belief and the attendant feelings are what need further clarification. If the therapist chose to go in the direction of talking about extroverts and introverts, she could have been distracted by the content, rather than digging for the possible emotion that was contained in the patient's initial statement. Talking about the difference between introverts and extroverts might have led to an interesting intellectual discussion, but it also runs the risk of moving away from understanding what triggered the patient's initial statement of not feeling connected to people.

As we continue to follow the dialogue, the therapist decided to address the patient's underlying assumptions, by asking if the patient automatically assumes that extroverts have an easier time knowing what to say. Here is where we discover what triggered the patient emotionally. The patient discloses that her friend said, *"I'm more of an open person, and you are more closed."* Clearly, the patient heard her friend's comment as a criticism and then tried to manage her fears around being judged by attributing her "shortcomings" to the fact that she was an introvert. This could serve the function of distancing from painful feelings by finding an intellectual explanation to hold onto. However, in the therapist's next statement, she continues to probe for the feeling underneath the surface by asking the patient how her friend's comment made her feel. It is at this point that the patient is then able to access a memory from high school, where her mother called her awkward and told her she didn't fit in. Mom labeled the patient's innate shyness as something that was wrong with her.

By tracking the dialogue in the present moment, we see how unfinished business from the past gets reactivated by present triggers. Here is how the use of entry point tracking allows the past to resurface without the therapist having to lead the client back to connections from early childhood. These memories often come up organically by tracking the phrases and emotions that are revealed when we use the patient's language to lead us.

Reviewing What Was Uncovered with the Client

The next template offers a format that directs the therapist to aspects of the dialogue that warrant further conversation. By reviewing the original exchange between the client and her friend, this allows the client to recognize the trigger point that led to possible erroneous assumptions she may have had made. This form of joint reflection and review allows for more of the client's feelings of vulnerability and shame to come to the surface. In this way the therapist can help to neutralize the patient's feelings of shame and refute mother's messages. Thus, further integration of the insights can be internalized around this disclosure.

You will note that at the top of the iceberg, we begin with the same entry point word or phrase that began the initial inquiry. This time, the therapist begins to clarify what is underneath the client's assumption, by repeating the phrase or asking what the client what she thinks it means. Avenues of exploration could include:

- connecting the patient's thoughts with attendant feelings or fears.
- asking what the patient did or said following the statement that triggered her.
- becoming curious about what made the client freeze up.

Once the initial entry point tracking uncovers a breakthrough in insight or memory retrieval, the therapist can then use this opportunity to go back and review with the client what she had learned from this dialogic exchange. In this case, the therapist begins with examining the assumptions that the client made when she heard the critical comment from her friend. The therapist then follows up by asking what the patient could have done to verbally check whether her assumption was accurate rather than automatically believing that it was true. This opens a further window of curiosity as a means of breaking the automatic, internalized reflex, where the client believed her mother's message actually reflected the truth about who she was (Figure 4.3).

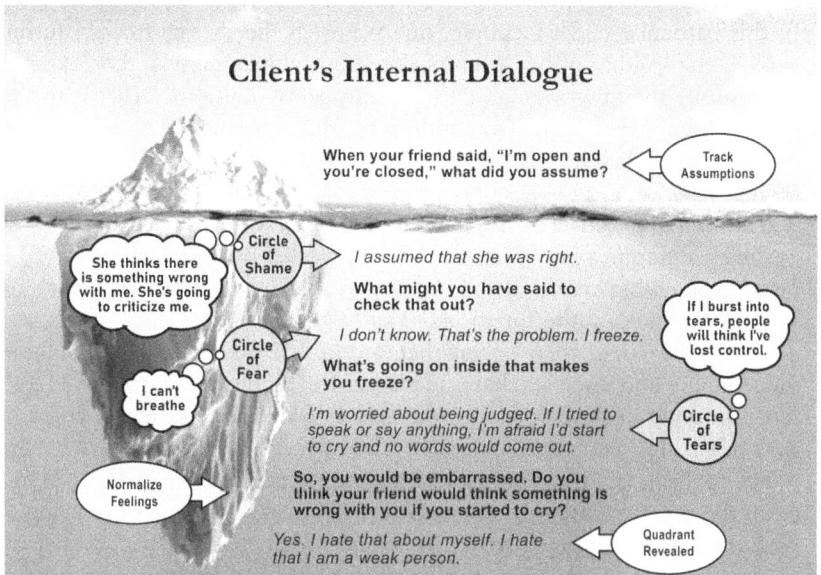

Figure 4.3 Client's Internal Dialogue.

We can also ask what might have been occurring on a body level that prevented the patient from asking for clarification from her friend. As you can see from the diagram, by focusing on bodily sensations and attending to what was happening physiologically, the patient was then able to remember that she couldn't breathe and that she was afraid she would burst into tears. For this patient, crying in front of another person was a shame trigger. The patient associated crying with losing control and thus assumed that her friend would negatively judge her for this. By paying attention to what the client is experiencing on a physical level as well as a cognitive level, this gives us an opportunity to access hidden shame. This not only integrates cognitive techniques with emotional triggers, it also connects somatic responses with beliefs and assumptions.

After this second exchange, the client was then able to articulate her buried or deeply-bound self-hatred around the belief that she is a weak person. In her family of origin losing control was forbidden, and this admission reveals where her feelings of self-loathing, contained in Quadrant Four, have been hidden. Admitting them out loud gives the therapist an opportunity to give reassurance in an effort to normalize her feelings and quiet the feelings of self-hate. Together, the therapist and the client could then explore the validity of these feelings, in hopes that the client will eventually be able to release the early internalized messages she had received from mother.

Taking the Entry Point Tracking Further

In this particular client example, one way that the therapist could further explore the validity of her assumptions about vulnerability and weakness is to continue the questioning. The diagram below illustrates what is further revealed about the client's assumptions as well as her beliefs about pressure, some of what has fueled her over-determined efforts in Quadrant One (Figure 4.4).

The therapist can take the entry-point process one step further by repeating a different phrase that the client revealed by wondering about her belief that crying makes her a weak person. She repeats the client's assumption by asking the question, *"You believe that crying makes you a weak person?"* The client then reveals her mother's reaction to her childhood vulnerability and discloses that it made her feel alone and worthless. Here is where deeper feelings of isolation and self-loathing begin to come to the surface. The patient then discloses the rules she has come to live by. She is not to have or show needs and she must strive to be perfect. At this point the therapist attempts to connect the patient's response of freezing up with the amount of pressure this must put on her. Rather than connecting to the therapist's reflection, the client reasserts her defensive strategy by stating that putting pressure on herself is what has made her achieve success in her career. It is with this revelation that we are able to better understand how the client's over-determined efforts in Quadrant One have been sustained by the positive reinforcement that a successful career has afforded

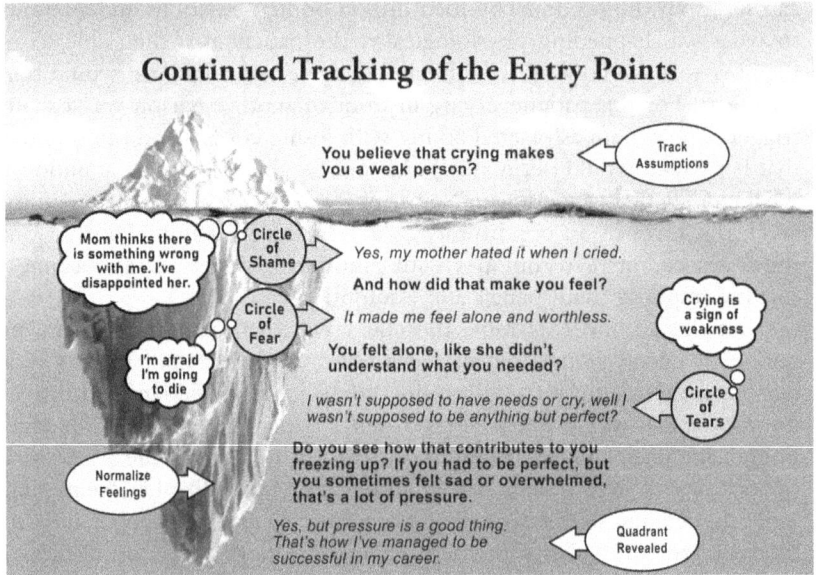

Figure 4.4 Continued Tracking of Entry Points.

her. It also enables the client to again shift away from her feelings of vulnerability. This is an indication to the therapist that she may need to tread more carefully and slow the inquiry process down a bit. Instead, the therapist decided to switch gears around further exploration as you will see in the next section.

Reflecting Current Insights and Practicing Alternative Sequences

Once the therapist registered that the client believed that feeling pressured was a positive attribute, she decided to back up and move toward where the client expressed a willingness to step out of her self-protective posture. The client had agreed that it would be a good idea to try to share more of her vulnerability with her friend. The therapist then chose to go back to the original entry point statement and begins her inquiry at the point where the client had involuntarily shut-down in a freeze response. The therapist asked what the client could have done as an alternative to freezing up. When clients are in a non-triggered state, asking what they could have done or wished they had done instead can create an opening for the client's own resilience and creative problem-solving to emerge.

In this case, the client volunteered that she could have asked her friend what she meant by the original statement in order to get further clarification. When the therapist encouraged the client to continue, she also volunteered that she could reveal more information to her friend around her fears of being judged. This then gave the therapist an opportunity to provide reassurance as well as to support the client's willingness to take a risk and step into more tender disclosure.

In the iceberg diagram below, notice that the client realizes that taking more of a risk would be a good thing in so far as it would allow her to stretch into exposing more of her vulnerability, trusting that it wouldn't result in shame or judgment. Utilizing entry point exploration as a means of creating new opportunities for behavioral change is one way that this technique can be a way of practicing new behavior without emotional triggers flooding cognitive processes. It is also a way that new organizing schematics can begin to be introduced along-side of deeply held assumptions and old memory tapes (Figure 4.5).

During all of the steps illustrated in each of the above diagrams, it is also important that we keep our attention fixed to how the patient is reacting to the dialogic exchange moment by moment. As Paul Wachtel (2011) states, "Effective inquiry increases the likelihood that the patient will experience the therapist's comments as an invitation to explore rather than take them as a challenge to be warded off or as a signal to hide." He further states that comments couched in the form of inquiries are sometimes interpreted by the client as having accusatory connotations and that the art of therapeutic

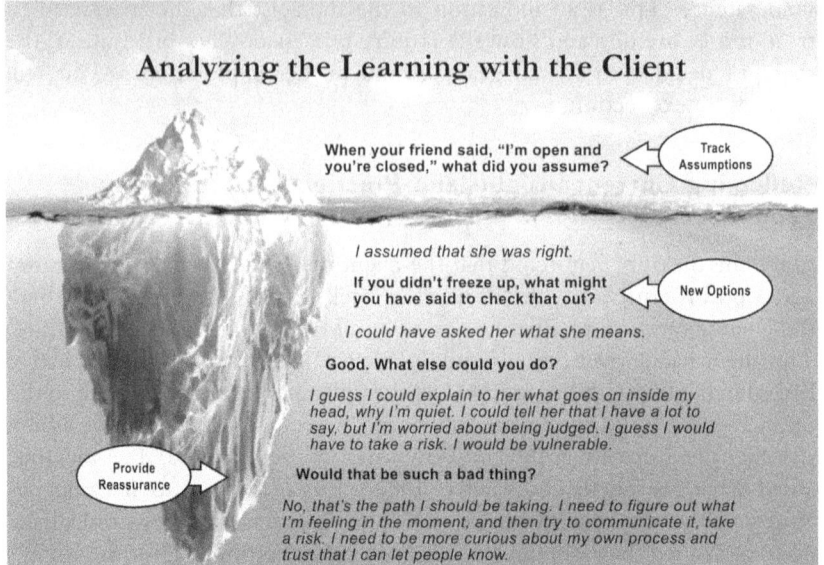

Figure 4.5 Analyzing the Learning with Clients.

inquiry is successfully demonstrated by leading the patient gently and gradually into territory that he has heretofore been afraid to face (p. 144).

If feelings of confusion, embarrassment, or defensiveness begin to surface, it is useful to provide some form of reassurance to normalize the patient's reactions and to help to manage and maintain affect regulation. It is also important to slow the process down, knowing that the material will resurface in future conversations. Through repeated efforts of slowing the process down and asking for clarification, clients are eventually able to understand what triggers their freeze response. Once this becomes conscious, clients are then able to release underlying feelings of shame that had remained under the surface.

A final step in working with entry point tracking is to provide the patient with opportunities to practice ways she could rehearse handling the conversation in the future. Again, in the following diagram (Figure 4.6), we begin with the initial entry point statement.

Here we see the patient taking charge of the dialogue by asking her friend for clarification about what she meant by her opening remark, *"I'm more open and you're more closed."* In doing so she is also asking her friend to clarify her own needs about what she is wanting from the friendship that she is possibly not getting. This question moves the dialogue away from accusation and into negotiation. It offers the opportunity for both to deepen the mutuality between them. It also allows the client to be freed up to share the reasons for her vulnerability, thus taking a step in the direction

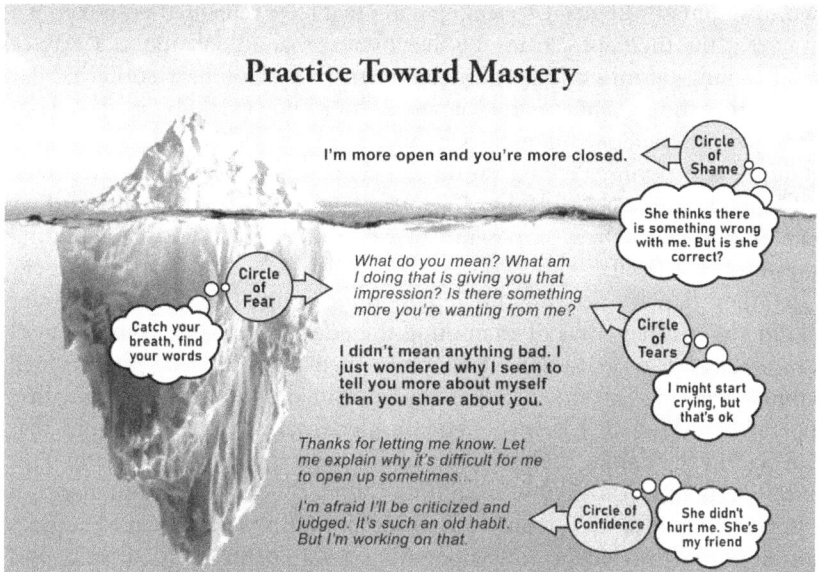

Figure 4.6 Practice Toward Mastery.

of proactive rather than reactive exchanges. This form of rehearsal brings cognitive/behavioral techniques into a fluid and organic psychodynamic framework, using rehearsal toward mastery in the context of the unfolding dialogic exchange between the therapist and client.

Summary

Using language as an entry point into deeper exploration not only helps therapists gain greater understanding of their clients, it eventually increases the patient's capacity for self-reflection, which in turn gradually leads to authentic self-emergence and increased resilience. Reflecting back what we heard and asking for clarification uses language as a discovery process, where the therapist gradually uncovers the particular nuances of each client's psychic organization. Furthermore, working with entry points is a way for us to recognize trigger points in the conversation that will lead us into deeper, unconscious material. Working with the dialogic process in this way allow us to be led by the client, which is far easier therapeutic position than trying push or to coax the client into an insight. Because of this, our clients will begin to feel held, respected, and seen. As trust deepens, clients will naturally begin to reveal what has been hidden, both from others and themselves.

When themes or patterns begin to emerge, the therapist can also "suggest" certain words or phrases, as a means of forecasting what might be just under consciousness, but not quite ready to emerge. Offering possible words or phrases language to feeling states that have remained unspoken is a way that the therapist can use his/her own verbal articulation as a way of telegraphing permission, as an encouragement to look at a corner of her world that the patient was told never to look. For example, in this client example the therapist might suggest that *pressure to be perfect* seems to be a double-edge sword. Picking up on the client's association that pressure is what made her successful, the therapist can open a doorway into further exploration as to the positive and negative aspects as a result of putting pressure on oneself.

Rather than confronting the defense directly, the therapist can wonder aloud about other ways of examining the effect of pressure. Once stated, the words linger in the air. Though pushed away at first, patients will come back to revisit the idea that was contained within this seed planting operation. Material that was once considered taboo, or assumptions that fell within the patient's blind spot, now have a chance to percolate. This form of permission-giving is another way an entry point can open a doorway that leads to unconscious material. In this way language becomes an intentional a seed-planting operation, a way of inviting curiosity and self-reflection rather than offering an interpretation that could evoke feelings of shame or resistance.

As Paul Wachtel (2011) reminds us, there are facilitative and non-facilitative ways to engage in a dialogic inquiry with our patients. He cautions, "Comments couched in the form of inquiries, like any other comments therapists make, are capable of having accusatory (or ex-culpatory) connotations. The art of inquiry in therapy is one of leading the patient gently and gradually into territory he has heretofore been afraid to face" (p. 144). This chapter has focused on working with entry points in a patient's language as a way of not only listening more carefully to our patients, but hopefully it has also provided guidance and clear clinical examples of ways that therapists can become more proficient at gently uncovering material that is too fearful for our patients to face.

References

Gianotti, P., & Danielian, J. (2017). *Uncovering the resilient core: A workbook on the treatment of narcissistic defenses, shame, and emerging authenticity.* Routledge.

Stern, D. B. (2015). *Relational freedom: Emergent properties of the relational field.* Routledge.

Wachtel, P. (2011). *Therapeutic communication: Knowing what to say when.* The Guilford Press.

5 Mastering the Technique of Moment-to-Moment Tracking: Mirroring, Sequential Reflection, and Reframing

Introduction

In Chapter Four, you were introduced to the concept of tracking entry points in language as a means of gaining greater clarity into words or phrases that patients use to disclose or mask their hopes, fears, assumptions, and relational expectation. Chapter Four also highlighted how the use of entry-point communication could be used as a means of getting beneath the tip of the iceberg to increase therapeutic listening and intervention skill sets. In this chapter, we will explore other examples of how to utilize moment-to-moment tracking to *mirror*, *synthesize*, and *integrate* patient material into a more cohesive narrative.

Moment-to-moment tracking is *how* we stay in the relational present. Too often when a patient reveals a comment that uncovers an emotion, therapists will either lead the patient forward to try to mitigate a negative feeling state, or they may go back in time to try to connect the emotion to a historical antecedent. Connecting the past to the present can be a powerful intervention strategy; however, if a therapist prematurely moves away from the present, a therapeutic rupture may occur. The art of moment-to-moment tracking, therefore, is a way we can capture the sequential unfolding of our clients' reactions and responses without trying to lead the client in a particular direction based on our own objectives or assumptions. It is how we can momentarily interrupt the conversational flow to gather more information about emotional triggers and reflexive thought patterns.

The technique of moment-to-moment tracking begins by identifying the entry point phrase that triggered an emotional reaction. Then, we attempt to walk our clients through the sequence of what occurred step-by-step. It is important to identify as many parts of the unfolding sequence as possible because often our clients are not consciously aware of how they arrived at their responses. Thoughts or assumptions that may have caused an escalation of feelings often remain out of the client's conscious awareness; or something in the therapeutic exchange may have triggered a micro-dissociative reaction that may go unregistered by either the client or

DOI: 10.4324/9781003120278-6

therapist. The technique of moment-to-moment tracking is a method of slowing the process down enough so that we are able to catch these reflexive triggers and bringing them into the shared, conscious dialogue between therapist and client.

Few clients have the ability to slow themselves down enough to be able to think about their reactions *before* they respond. For example, a client may say, "*I got a call from my ex-boyfriend and before I knew it, I was screaming at him on the phone, calling him a loser and a jerk. This happens every time he calls. I can't seem to stop myself, and I feel so foolish afterwards. He has such a way of getting under my skin.*" The underlying assumption contained within this statement is that the patient believes she has no control over her emotions when it comes to her ex-boyfriend. This assumption shuts down her curiosity as to what happens between them sequentially that invariably culminates in the same reaction.

If we were to utilize the technique of moment-to-moment tracking in this situation, we would begin by asking the patient to go back and try to track the details of what occurred within the sequence of the phone call to help her learn how to manage her reactivity. For example, we could ask:

- What happened when you picked up the phone and realized it was your ex?
- What thoughts or feelings did you have when you first heard his voice?
- Do you remember the first thing he said to you?
- How did that make you feel?
- What did you say in response?
- When do you remember starting to get irritated?
- Did any other thoughts pop into your mind when you first noticed your irritation?
- What do you wish you had said instead?

These questions, listed sequentially, help patients learn how to identify thought or feeling triggers that may have gone unnoticed when reactivity quickly escalates. In this case walking through the details of the event can actually model for the patient how to slow her own process down in order that she can prepare her responses differently the next time the ex-boyfriend calls.

When patients begin to notice more of the details around the sequence of their thoughts, this is how their response patterns can be interrupted. The therapist begins by initiating questions that illuminate unconscious or unregistered parts of the patient's reactions. Often patients will remember forgotten details of an unfolding sequence when you slow the inquiry process down and ask them to review what happened step by step. Sequential tracking is also a way of co-regulating affect by catching emotional trigger-points that then enable the patient's cognitive processing to be brought back online. In other words, sequential tracking is one way to help patients move out of a hyper-aroused state, shifting from habituated, reflexive responses to a state where cognitions and feelings can work in concert.

The same is true when it comes to catching patterns where patients move into hypo-aroused states. When the sympathetic nervous system is overloaded by feelings of shame or disgust, or when the experience of the safety within the therapeutic alliance is broken, patients with insecure attachment histories may experience a micro-dissociative shut-down. For example, the therapist may make an interpretation that exposes something outside of the patient's awareness, thus triggering feelings of shame. Or, if a therapist questions the patient in an attempt to understand his/her anxiety response, the very nature of the questions may trigger a dissociative shut-down.

Not knowing when and how to push a client in ways that remain affectively tolerable is generally where therapeutic missteps often occur. Lichtenberg (2001) states that in order to appreciate a patient's motivation we need to discern their emotional experience, and at times that will be difficult to uncover. He states, "The golden thread in assessing motivation lies in discovering the affect being sought in conjunction with the behavior being investigated" (p. 444). Watching for trigger points that then lead to a sequence of reactions is the way in which we unravel that "golden thread" that allows the therapist to detect the underlying emotion that may be driving a patient's thoughts or behaviors. Once we have a better grasp of the patient's underlying emotions and/or assumptions, we are then in a better position to help calm the nervous system and bring them back into their window of tolerance. This also reestablishes the patient's connection with the therapist in the present moment.

Once the patient is re-regulated, the therapist and patient can explore thoughts, feelings, and assumptions that may have triggered the dissociative shut-down. It is in these moments that the therapist then has an opportunity to reframe old, negative assumptions that often accompany painful feelings in a way that allows the patient to feel a greater sense of self-agency as well as a decreased feeling of shame. Wachtel (2011) states, "It is often in the patient's 'framing' of the truth, in the particular way he organizes, categorizes, and gives emotional meaning to what has transpired, that his difficulty lies. And it is the therapist's new and different—and generally less accusatory—framing of the truth that can open the possibility for cure" (p. 124).

It is important to remember that the simple act of asking a series of questions to gather more information may be experienced as a challenge to some patients. Patients with a hypervigilant fear response may be triggered into a hypo-arousal shut down if they feel bombarded by too many questions. These shutdowns may be quite subtle and may initially remain undetected by the therapist. For example, one patient eventually revealed, "I learned to disappear when my father would bombard me with his questions. It was the only way I could stay safe, the only way he couldn't catch me in a mistake." When asked if the therapist's questions ever triggered a similar shut-down, the patient replied, "Sometimes." Thus, the unfolding inquiry process can trigger a breach in the patient's feeling of connection and safety at any moment. And yet, all therapists must proceed into areas that will eventually trigger some degree of patient discomfort. Bromberg (2006) reminds us that the therapeutic relationship must feel safe, but not perfectly safe. Walking that fine line is not always easy. However, if we observe a sympathetic nervous-system shut-down, we can recover and reconnect with the patient by going back to the moment of rupture and repair what occurred. This form of repair in the present moment can reestablish the relational connection and strengthen trust in the therapeutic alliance.

In summary, moment-to-moment tracking is the essence and the "glue" of therapeutic conversation. As we stay firmly focused in the present moment, a picture slowly begins to emerge, revealing where pockets of pain are deeply hidden, where early wishes and longings remain, and where over-determined efforts attempt to hide feelings of loneliness, and disenfranchisement. Gradually, we also begin to hear where glimmers of authenticity come through in statements that seem to contradict old patterns and beliefs. It is in these moments that we are able to see their innocence and unblemished decency, their raw talents and gifts beginning to be verbalized. It is only by remaining steady in this diligent and persistent tracking process that we can grasp how pockets of shame or feelings of inadequacy are being sequestered. And once released, the authentic self has permission and access to emerge.

Moment-to-Moment Tracking as a Form of Reflection, Naming, and Connecting Parts of the Patient's Narrative to Other Parts

The technique of moment-to-moment tracking can be used to increase the patient's self-reflective capacities through simply *naming* what might be just under the surface of conscious awareness. As the therapist listens for repeated patterns and/or points of confusion, s/he can then respond with his/her own reflections as a means of clarifying, and/or normalizing the patient's conflict. This technique can also be used to integrate disavowed parts of the patient's psyche into the existing conscious narrative. This is particularly true when the therapist searches for ways in which s/he can challenge over-determined efforts that have become habitually self-destructive.

In the following section two client examples will be provided that illustrate how naming a particular conflict or behavioral pattern can be used to interrupt habituated thought processes. The first case vignette illustrates an exchange between a patient and therapist where the therapist continues to ask clarifying questions. Although this is initially useful as a means of gathering important information, at some point reflecting or reframing what the therapist heard helps patients more clearly see their underlying conflict or their defensive response patterns. The second client example illustrates how naming the behavioral sequence aloud helps to reveal the patient's distorted, self-destructive assumptions. Both case vignettes reflect typical exchanges that often occur between therapists and clients, one's that may lead to a power struggle or therapeutic impasse.

Client Example One

Client: *It feels like I need help thinking through some conflicts that are happening and creating tensions. I am wrestling with these daily. One has to do with Larry, my partner, and the other my own needs and understanding of things I'm feeling pulled towards... like my destiny.*

Therapist: *Ok. What are the conflicts that are creating the tensions?*

Client: *I feel like the tensions revolve around how I see myself in the center of my relationship with Larry. His posture feels so entitled. As things come up, he texts me, fires things off. He constantly texts me questions like "Who is the first person you think of in the morning?" or "Will you ever love me again." Or "How much longer should I wait for you." I just want to drive far away. I feel trapped and I get very flustered. I know what he's trying to do: it's entrapment. No matter what I say I'll be in trouble. Sometimes I think I don't want a relationship at all right now. I need to step back and look at myself in an honest way.*

Therapist: *Sounds like it is creating a lot of stress. Would walking away be a way of escaping what you are feeling?*

Client: *I want space to think about myself.*

Therapist: *What does that look like?*

Client: *Being able to put the relationship on hold. Being in charge of my own wants and desires, my schedule, to be the owner of my own time. It is like I constantly need to be there for him. It is hard to discover myself. Time doesn't feel like my own.*

Therapist: *Is it like you feel like you don't have a choice?*

Client: *It is like I can't set boundaries. If I'm Larry's emotional outlet, the one he leans on, then it is hard to say no.*

Therapist: *Does that remind you of your mother?*

Client: *No, my mother isn't that pushy. I'm talking about Larry. I just want my freedom.*

Therapist: *Ok, what might happen if you said no, if you let Larry know you were unable to be there for him right now?*

Client: *Larry is so tightly wound. If he hears I'm not going to do such and such or commit...it is all seen as an affront or a threat, like I'm cutting him off, that I'm not being open or honest. It is easier not to say anything.*

Analysis

The client presents with a complaint, and the therapist asks a series of questions, wondering what makes the patient feel stuck, unable to set a limit. The therapist then suggests a connection to the patient's past history with her mother, and the patient denies that this might be a similar struggle, in spite of the fact that the patient has complained about feeling trapped by her mother's tight rein in previous sessions. The therapist then shifts her questioning to focus on what might happen if the patient were able to say "no" to Larry. The patient quickly shifts away from herself and back to describing how Larry would respond. Her solution is to assume a passive position, claiming *"it is easier not to say anything."* We can imagine that the therapist might then ask, "How is that easier?" And we can also imagine the patient giving a justification why that would be so.

At some point in the exchange, it might be useful to simply make a reflective comment, one that articulates the patient's conflict. For example, the therapist could say, *"So, let me see if I understand your struggle. There is a part of you that wants to be in charge of your own needs and desires, to be the owner of your time, but when you're with someone who makes demands on you, you give into their needs? Is that correct? I wonder what happens to your desire for freedom in those moments – those times when someone is asking something from you?"* This type of reflective comment, naming the two sides of the conflict followed by a question that directs the patient to the moment she loses sight of herself, can often help the client pause and begin to wonder just what it is that allows her to give up on herself and give into the demands of another.

Notice that this type of statement doesn't pull the client in any direction (toward making a connection to her struggle with her mother or thinking about the possibility of setting a limit with Larry.) It simply allows the client to hear the two sides of her struggle repeated out loud. Hearing another person put your conflict into words often allows a person to be more fully seen and understood. The follow-up question is then able to help the client notice where and how she loses sight of herself. Once this occurs, the therapist and client can join in becoming more curious as to how and why this happens. Underlying fears are then likely to come to the surface and shared verbally, rather than the patient's fears remaining unconscious as she maintains a stance of passive frustration. Once our patients are able to articulate their fears to a trusted other, they are likely to feel less isolated or confused by their seeming inability to take action.

In this client example an alternative way to name the patient's struggle would be to directly speak to the partner's behavior as you, the therapist, imagine that the patient is actually experiencing it. For example, the patient says that Larry is demanding, entitled, and trying to trap her. The therapist might reframe the partner's behavior as aggressive, even bordering on coercive. The therapist could wonder out loud asking, *"How many people fire off 20–30 texts a day when you've clearly asked for space? That must feel suffocating."* Naming the partner's behavior in this way gives the patient permission to own and validate her feelings as reasonable. It is also a way of speaking "in between the lines" to the underlying loyalty contract that originally made it taboo to speak out against an overly controlling parent. Working with a loyalty contract in the derivative by using this patient's enactment with her partner can set the stage for further exploration into issues of fairness and relational expectations that manifest as repeated patterns in Quadrant Three.

Client Example Two

In this next client example, a patient who suffers from chronic pain speaks to her therapist about being disappointed with herself as measured by *"giving in"* and taking her pain medication. She feels ashamed and inadequate for having chronic pain, and when the pain flares up, she often goes to a dark place where she feels suicidal and hopeless, telling herself that *"the pain won."* The patient disclosed that when she was a child, her parents ignored a back injury she suffered from, telling her that it was all in her head and that she was a baby, whining and trying to get attention. She remembers that she made a vow to show them that she wasn't weak by pushing through the pain and ignoring it. Now, in the present when she experiences a pain flare-up, she becomes angry and calls herself weak. However, she is unable to see the connection between how her parents treated her in the past and her internalized associations to her pain in the present. The repeated cycle of behavior during the course of her therapy is illustrated in the following diagram. Figure 5.1

This diagram illustrates a vicious cycle that is fueled by over-determined efforts to resist feelings of shame and inadequacy that she has come to associate with having a painful illness. Part of her belief system is that it is her fault that she is in pain as we can see reflected in some of her statements to the therapist below. She sees it as a battle that she must win to prove her self-worth, prove that she is stronger than the pain. Her strategy is to initially resist her pain by trying to distract herself with busy work or manual tasks. At times she can feel the pain diminish, and she feels proud of her ability to overcome the pain. This reenforces her belief that this strategy can work. However, when the therapist attempts to penetrate her belief system, asking the patient what would happen if she let herself rest or if she allowed herself to take medication before the pain intensified, the patient would respond with statements such as:

> *I just want my life back.*
> *I can't let the pain win. I'm better than this.*
> *I need to psyche myself up to get used to the pain.*
> *I'm not interested in resting; I need to get stuff done.*
> *I've always been this way; I like to push myself. It makes me feel strong.*
> *It feels like you're trying to get me to take the easy way out. I don't want to be weak.*
> *I'm trying to do my best.*
> *I'm a God-fearing woman, there must be something wrong with me.*
> *Am I being punished for not doing enough? Is that why the pain keeps coming back.*

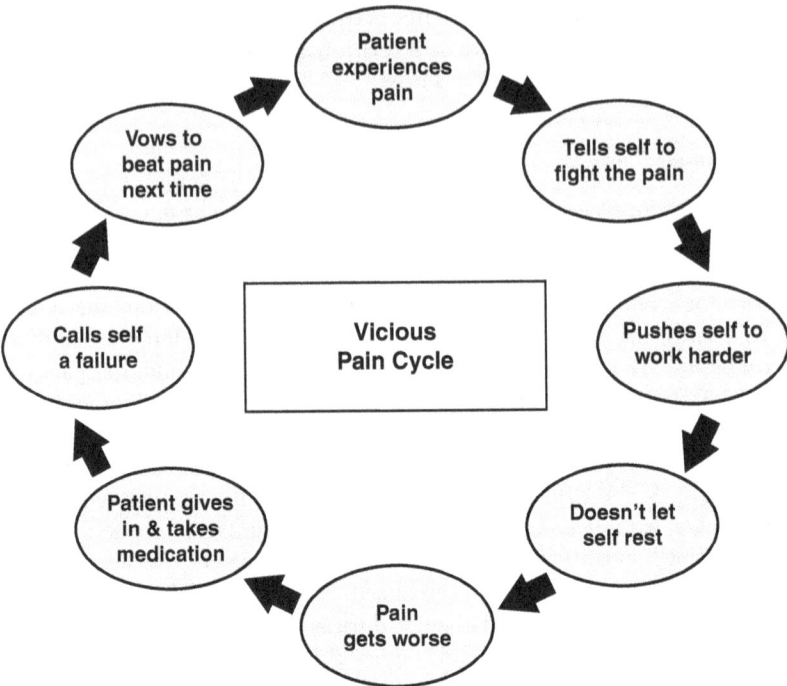

Figure 5.1 Vicious Pain Cycle.

Whenever the therapist tried to question the patient's harsh standards in Quadrant One, the patient would come back with one of the above responses. Notice that the patient's comments about why the pain is happening is as if a harsh parent is punishing her for doing something wrong. This harsh standard remains unquestioned, normalized by the belief that the act of pushing herself is what actually makes her feel stronger.

When the therapist tried to empathize with the patient's frustration and disappointment, the patient would become even more adamant in her need to not show weakness. The therapist felt that it was impossible to find an entry point into breaking the defensively based pattern. It felt as if they were in a tug of war. In a consultation session it was suggested that it may be useful to speak to both sides of the conflict simultaneously, to reflect back the sequence of events as the thoughts seemed to unfold in the patient's mind. An example of how this reflection process could occur is as follows:

1. *It seems as though that whenever you have a pain flare-up, you get angry and try to resist the need to take medication.*
2. *Then you tell yourself that you should be able to overcome the pain. Or you tell yourself that you need to get used to the pain.*
3. *And you then push yourself into work, trying to ignore the pain. You don't let yourself rest.*
4. *Invariably the pain gets worse. When the pain gets too intense, you give in and take the medication.*
5. *And even though the pain goes away, you tell yourself that the pain won. And that thought makes you feel defeated, even suicidal. But you vow to yourself that you'll beat the pain next time.*
6. *It doesn't seem that this strategy is working very well, and yet you keep trying it over and over again.*
7. *Do you think that we can look at this sequence together and come up with some different strategies that won't leave you feeling defeated or suicidal?*

Reflecting the entire sequence back to the client followed by the observation that the patient's strategy isn't working, often creates an opening where the patient can consciously acknowledge that her strategy isn't working. With this acknowledgement, hopefully the patient's own curiosity and self-reflective capacities will be activated. Verbally declaring (naming) the fact that the patient's strategy isn't working bring aspects of reality into the conversation to help penetrate the over-determined wish that she could conquer her physical pain by sheer will-power. Finally, asking for permission to try something new can dismantle the patient's learned/automatic response to pain. This form of tracking the sequence by *reflecting, naming, and asking permission* often breaks through the defensive posture that manifests in enactments or struggles that often come up between therapists and clients.

As you will notice, there are many of the patient's assumptions that could be followed up on by using them as entry-points into further exploration. However, remaining in the moment, giving the patient permission to accept the fact that the pain is not her fault, can be a grounding experience, a shift toward gentleness and self-care. Asking the patient for permission to join with the therapist to try to deal with her pain in a more compassionate way can also be a moment where the patient can feel connected to a helpful other. She no longer has to be fighting through the pain alone, the condition she was left in by her parents during childhood.

Tracking Sequential Patterns in Couples Therapy

This section will illustrate how moment-to-moment tracking can be a useful tool in helping couples reestablish productive communication patterns. Often couples get lost in the content of a disagreement when trying to prove a point or win an argument. Power struggles can disguise underlying emotions that have become activated due to fear or shame. Sequentially tracking the exact words of the conversational sequence, as well as asking about underlying thoughts or feelings that weren't been expressed verbally, can present a clearer picture as to how emotional triggers become activated. Once the underlying thoughts or feelings are brought into conscious awareness, the therapist can suggest to the couple that it is beneficial and clarifying to let their partner know the thoughts and feelings that are being triggered in the moment. Sharing the parts of the self that are being triggered by old memories or associations can actually deescalate the situation in the present moment and increase a sense of compassion for each other.

The following client example illustrates how differing expectations as to how to approach a minor household chore can escalate into feelings of devaluation and shame. In this case I will refer to our couple discussed in Chapter Two, Kathy and Ben, where issues of shame and devaluation were active trigger points in their communication patterns with each other. This specific vignette centers on the friction caused by who does the laundry. Struggles over the laundry had been an unresolved sore point since the beginning of their marriage. Although the couple was able to deescalate more quickly after this most recent fight about the laundry, their ability to process why this issue continued to be a sticking point remained a mystery to them.

When asked to walk through the conversation, we were able to identify a negative assumption on Kathy's part that led to her feel angry and frustrated with Ben. Kathy assumed that Ben was taking advantage of her because he waited until laundry piled up knowing that it bothered her. She reported that because of her frustration she gave in and ended up doing the laundry the majority of the time. She believed Ben was intentionally dragging his feet, which in turn triggered her anger. The conversational sequence is as follows:

Kathy: *"Just because you're fine wearing dirty clothes, doesn't mean I am. Why don't you help with the laundry rather than waiting for me to do it?"*

Ben: *Whoa, wait a minute. I never wear dirty clothes, what are you talking about? That's not fair."*

Kathy: *But I'm always the one doing the laundry. I'm sick of waiting for you to do it and having all those dirty clothes pile up."*

Ben: *I don't wear dirty clothes. When did you ever see me wear dirty clothes? I may change into work clothes when I'm in the yard, but they're never dirty.*

Kathy: (*Withdraws for a few moments, and then says.*) *Ok, I'm sorry. I shouldn't have said that. I apologize. Let's just forget about it.*

Ben: *No, I want to talk about it. I don't understand why you said that? Where's that coming from?*

Kathy: *I said I'm sorry. What more do you want from me?*

Ben: *I want to know what made you say that. Do you really think I'm a slob? Look, I do the laundry too. I just wait until it piles up and then do it all at once. Not like you, you like to do laundry every day.*

Kathy: *Ok, ok. Let's just let this go. I said I'm sorry.*

When we processed this sequence, the couple did say that they thought they had made progress in comparison to conversations in years past. First, Kathy realized that she had been triggered because she made an assumption that Ben was taking advantage of her. Rather than sharing her assumption, she lashed out with a criticism. However, she immediately realized she had made a mistake and apologized. She stated that in the past, she would never apologize; she would just withdraw. Ben agreed that the apology was better than the silent treatment; however, he still wanted to know where the comment was coming from. When he pressed for answers, Kathy felt that her apology wasn't good enough. She then felt that Ben had moved into lecture-mode and that he was trying to humiliate her for lashing out in the first place. At this point Kathy had a memory flashback of sitting in a rocking chair when she was a little girl and having her mother lecture her for her wrongdoing.

What is interesting is that both parties in this exchange felt victimized. Both felt that they were trying to exercise new behavior, and neither felt that their partner fully understood that they were making an effort to try to understand/to try to make amends. The following two diagrams illustrate how each party felt misunderstood and somewhat victimized by the other. Figure 5.2

Kathy's new insights had to do with recognizing how she could often lash out at Ben when she felt unsafe or devalued. This behavior was similar to what she witnessed her mother do to her when she was a child. Kathy reflected that her comment to Ben about wearing dirty clothes just slipped out before she could edit her thoughts. She told both the therapist and Ben that she regretted her comment the minute she said it; she was filled with feelings of embarrassment and shame. Prior to therapy, she was unable to make the connection that her behavior was similar to her mother's. Instead, she would focus on her assumption being true, giving her justification to withdraw as both a self-protective action and punishment to Ben. However, given her progress in therapy, Kathy was now able to catch herself and apologize. Because she was able to demonstrate this new behavior, she felt she deserved credit for trying to rectify the situation. Therefore, she became puzzled when Ben insisted on trying to process why she said what she said. She thought to herself, wasn't her

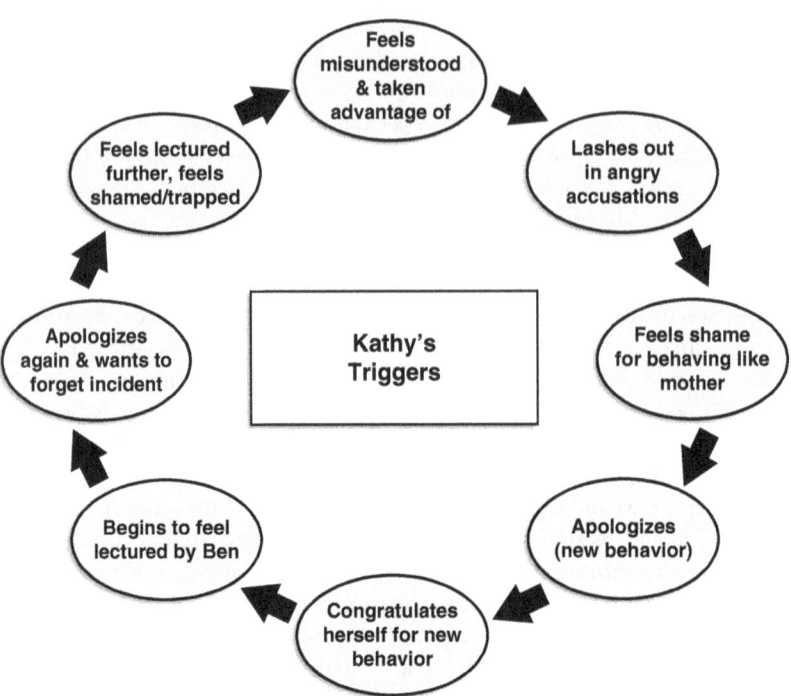

Figure 5.2 Kathy's Triggers.

apology seen as an improvement? Why couldn't he acknowledge that? Instead, she was being lectured to by Ben and felt that he was trying to make her suffer, rubbing her face in her mistake. Upon further reflection, she was then able to identify how her mother would often scream at her, lecturing her for what she had done wrong. After the diatribe, her mother would then act as if nothing had happened, wanting to move on without talking about it. Kathy, at that moment realized that she was doing the same thing to Ben.

In this next diagram we notice the cycle that is set into motion within Ben once Kathy lashed out at him. Not understanding where Kathy's comment was coming from, Ben feels wrongly accused and stays focused on the content of her comment trying to explain himself. Although Kathy's apology feels like an improvement, better than her withdrawal and distancing that occurred in the past, Ben is still confused by what her comment really means. He doesn't believe it really has to do with the laundry. His assumptions take him in the direction that she is dissatisfied with him in some deeper way, that her mistrust of him runs deeper than any gains that they have achieved in the therapy. As a way of distancing himself from his own feelings of hopelessness, he attempts to use logic, explaining himself to

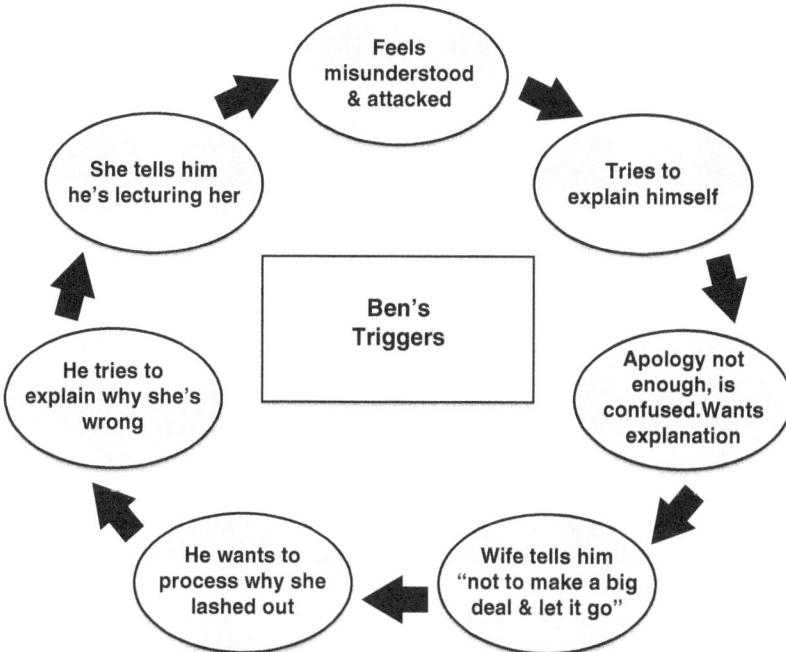

Figure 5.3 Ben's Triggers.

win Kathy's trust. This, in turn, triggers Ben's vicious cycle, where the use of intellect and logic are meant to convince someone that they are wrong, a behavior that is similar to what his father did to him. Figure 5.3

It was important for the therapist to find a way to break into these self-perpetuating cycles of misunderstanding and disconnect. When the therapist was able to track the underlying emotions that were being triggered during each phase of the conversational exchange, both Kathy and Ben were more able to see each other's triggers. For example, when Kathy was able to share out loud that she regretted her initial comment and felt like she was behaving like her mother, this allowed Ben to understand that Kathy's comment was reflexive – the residue of an old behavioral pattern when Kathy believed she was being undervalued. When the therapist asked Ben if it would have made a difference if Kathy had shared her feelings aloud that she felt ashamed for behaving like her mother, he said that it would make a huge difference. He would have been brought into her internal processing of the event, and he felt that he wouldn't have to keep justifying himself. Instead, he could be there for Kathy to help her feel less triggered by her shame. He stated that he could then also acknowledge to her that it made a big difference to him that she was able to apologize and not withdraw.

Remaining connected to each other during temporary moments of fracture – by sharing aloud underlying thoughts and feelings is one of the ways to move through the emotional tangle of triggering comments that lead to the fear of disconnection. When each person shares his/her internal thoughts as they are occurring, this can help clarify and cut through the isolation and the attendant shame and/or confusion when conversational ruptures occur. In this way each person can move to understanding and regain empathy for one another. It is a way to break through the vicious cycle of disconnected communication in a couple's system.

Using Moment–to–Moment Tracking to Enhance Mutual Recognition and Mirroring

Without verbal acknowledgement, without the mirroring response of mutual cuing of the serve and return of relational dialogue, unacknowledged aspects of the self will remain unknown or unformulated. As Harry Stack Sullivan (1953) reminds us, "One has information about one's experience only to the extent that one has tended to communicate it to another or thought about it in the manner of communicative speech. Much of that which is ordinarily said to be repressed is merely unformulated" (p. 185). Language is one of the primary therapeutic vehicles that convey the recognition of other. It takes the mirroring response of another to bring these vague tendencies into clearer view.

The need for personal recognition is an innate desire in every human being, one that is present from birth. If an infant is not sufficiently recognized, through mutual cuing and mirroring, the capacity to develop a solid sense of self, the capacity for mutuality in relationship, and the capacity to achieve ethical self-consciousness is thwarted. With the discovery of two large-scale mirroring neural networks that represent the self and others, the importance of mirroring and recognition theory have been validated and verified scientifically (Uddin et al., 2007). This section explores the various nuances of mirroring responses, and how the mirroring process leads to the development of the capacity for mutual recognition. Using moment-to-moment tracking as a means of therapeutic mirroring is not only a way to anticipate another person's intentions and resonate with their emotions, but also a way to create right-brain-to-right-brain resonance.

Repeated mirroring over time builds an earned, secure attachment within the parameters of the therapeutic relationship. As the treatment process unfolds, one important dimension of mirroring is the therapist's ability to catch early signs of change, moments in session when the client tentatively begins to test new ways of expressing self in relationship. This can take the form of increased insight, curiosity, or increased self-reflective capacities. Being able to notice and reflect these authentic aspects of self-expression back to the client as they emerge within the treatment hour is a way that new organizing schemas are built within the psyche.

Jessica Benjamin, along with the scientific validation from infant researchers, states that the act of mutual recognition encompasses a broad number of experiences that can be identified as emotional attunement, mutual influence, affective mutuality, and sharing states of mind. She states, "Recognition as an organizing idea may be thought of in two ways: First, as a psychic position in which we know the other's mind as an equal source of intention and agency, affecting and being affected: and second as a process or action, the essence of responsiveness in interaction" (2018, p. 3). Acts of recognition confirm to the patient that what they are saying, how they are presenting themselves are being seen by the therapist, and that their history and their intentions have been understood and held within the context of the holding relationship.

Furthermore, clients need to feel that who they are as a unique human being has an impact and that they matter to you as a therapist. They need to feel both connection and reliance on a trusted other, as well as experiencing the ability to assert oneself is the foundation of mutuality in relationship. Again, Benjamin (1988) states, "Assertion and recognition constitute the poles of a delicate balance. This balance is integral to what is called *differentiation*, the individual's development as a self that is aware of its distinctness from others. Yet this balance, and with it the differentiation of self and other, is difficult to sustain. In particular, the need for recognition gives rise to a paradox. Recognition is that response from the other which makes meaningful the feelings, intentions, and actions of the self" (p. 12). The ability to be seen and recognized comes from mirroring responses from a trusted other. Here is how differentiation of the self develops alongside a growing capacity for mutuality or mutual recognition in adult relationships.

Much of our personal narrative is shaped by external directives or cultural messages. They become part of the organizing schemas that comprise the foundation of character formation (Danielian & Gianotti, 2012, p. 21). As stated in Chapter One, organizing schemas are the unconscious and consciously constructed expectations of self and other as they relate to one's narrative, symptom presentation, level of trust, behavioral interactions, and the degree of relational connection or disconnection with others. Created in childhood to establish some semblance of safety and stability, defensively constructed schematics are limiting insofar as aspects of the authentic self were reflexively split off in order to maintain a precarious parental attachment. Louis DeRosis (1974) talks about how organizing schemas develop, and he describes this as an internalization process of the "insistent influence around us." D. W. Winnicott (1965) speaks of the disruptive impact of chronic empathic failures when he observed, "Often, the environmental factor is not a single trauma but a pattern of distorting influences; the opposite, in fact, of the facilitating environment which allow for individual maturation" (p. 139).

In childhood chronic and repeated messages are accepted as a "given." As people move into adulthood, many of their beliefs, values, and thought processes largely remain underexamined throughout their lives. This is particularly true for individuals who were taught that their opinion didn't matter, where it was unsafe or somehow wrong to challenge authority figures, or there was little interest in or attention given to the child's developing self. When these children reach adulthood, their communication style is rather concrete, conceptualizations are generally framed in black and white terms, and their interior world reflects little capacity for insight, where thoughts are poorly formulated, and where there is a general absence of curiosity about the larger world stage. The emotional dimension of self (one's emotional intelligence) often remains limited as well. Individuals with insecure attachment histories often display either a high level of reactivity on one end of the spectrum, or a blunting of effect on the other. Emotions are relatively undifferentiated, where individuals have difficulty expressing a range of feeling states; they are unable to differentiate one emotion from the next, or they are easily dysregulated by their emotions, where reflexive reactivity overpowers cognition.

One's internalized relational schematic does not remain fixed throughout the life span; rather, schemas can be altered by experiences and significant adult relationships, including the therapeutic relationship. What is quite hopeful is that the quality of one's relational attachment in the present can alter beliefs, perceptions, and experiences that comprise the organizing schema. This is why attention to language is important. How one listens to and tracks the flow of communication, stopping to clarify words or phrases, can be used as a therapeutic tool to gain deeper insight into a client's inner world. By attending to the details of language, by searching for what is being expressed *behind* the words themselves is what allows clients to feel seen and acknowledged in ways they had yet been able to recognize.

The following process recording illustrates how mirroring responses can help the patient feel that he is seen and understood, even when he struggles to put something into words. Mirroring responses help to bring less formulated reactions into a shared verbal/relational realm. As this patient talks to his therapist, we notice signs of newly emerging insights as he tries to connect his feelings to triggering events that make him feel overwhelmed. The therapist then mirrors the self-reflective capacities that are emerging, even though the client continues to feel overwhelmed by the external situation in the theater. This mirroring of increased capacity helps the patient internalize his feelings even further. The comments that are bolded and in parenthesis show where that the client is exhibiting gains in his capacity for self-regulation.

Client Illustration

Th: *Do you find that you've been able to track your thoughts more clearly when that feeling of chaos starts bubbling up?*

Pt: *Umm, I feel like I've been able to track my feelings more; I don't know about my thoughts. I just notice that I was feeling very overwhelmed. When people started pushing and were getting aggressive wanting to leave the theatre right then and there, I just felt myself getting overwhelmed.* (**Pt. is demonstrating an increased capacity to self-reflect rather than move into reflexive dissociation.**)

Th: *Mmm hmm.*

Pt: *So I walked to the back and sat down for a few minutes to try to calm myself.* (**Shows he has been able to strategize about self-care.**)

Th: *You were aware of the pressure that was building in your body, but it was hard to catch your thinking mind shutting down a little bit?*

Pt: *Yeah, it was just very... yeah, I guess I wasn't able to keep track of all the thoughts. It was very... just out of focus.* (**Starts to struggle for words.**)

Th: *Yes, but do you see that when you start to get overwhelmed rather than just shutting down, you were able to take care of yourself. You sat down for a minute in the theater to calm yourself down. That's pretty amazing. You weren't able to do that before. Even though you couldn't track all of your thoughts in that moment, you knew enough to sit down.* (**Therapist tracks the sequence and reaffirms this gain.**)

Pt: *Mmm, hmm, yeah, I guess you're right. I didn't think it was that big of a deal at the time, but it did help me calm down.* (**Some internalization of insights and acknowledgement of his progress**).

Th: *So as we go on, I think that's just something we can do – to slow down and try to track your thoughts, just like we have before with the feelings. (Pause) Are you aware of what made you think about wanting to take a break, sit down, and cool down?* (**Therapist attempts to connect thoughts to feelings and observations.**)

Pt: *I mean, I was very overwhelmed and I was, umm, I don't know. I don't know what I was thinking, it was a really weird situation. But I do remember looking at the person standing next to me, and she looked really nervous, and I thought to myself – well, I guess I'm not the only one. I guess that made me feel normal, and when I said that to myself, I was able to think about what I could do to calm the situation down.* (**Pt. remembers more of the unfolding sequence of his processing in the moment.**)

Th: *See, you were able to think something through. You used what you had registered about the person standing next to you as a way to reassure yourself that your feelings were normal. That seemed to calm you down enough to bring the thinking part of your mind back online – you were able to come up with a strategy to remove yourself from the chaos.* (**Reaffirmation and mirroring.**)

Analysis

This short vignette demonstrates how insight begins to emerge as the patient attempts to reflect and track the unfolding sequence of what happened at the very moment that he began to feel overwhelmed in the theater. In the past the patient would have dissociated and only a vague recollection of what happened would remain because he would have become flooded with feeling. As the patient recounts what occurred, he appears as if he has forgotten parts of the sequence. As the therapist encourages him to walk through what happened step-by-step, the patient is then able to remember more of his unfolding thoughts and reactions. In each instance of re-membering more of the details the therapist mirrors these details back to the patient as a means of helping the patient consciously connect more and more parts of the sequence together. This back-and-forth mirroring and tracking process enables the patient to gain further insight as well as internalize what he was able to accomplish in terms of self-care and affect regulation.

Part of what is involved in the mirroring response is facilitating memory retrieval by helping the patient connect parts with other parts of an unfolding sequence. This identification and connection of parts of the sequence to the whole experience helps build upon the client's ability to create a verbal narrative that describes the event more accu-rately. Rather than the theater event remaining an overwhelming experience, applying the technique of moment-to-moment tracking by using mirroring comments enables the client to hold onto his ex-perience with a sense of clarity and self-agency. In addition, the therapist is able to reframe the entire experience as a success, reflecting that the patient was able to accomplish something he had yet to ac-complish in the past. Over time, this type of mirroring response helps to lay in new neural pathways that assist in both the management of affect regulation as well as the ability to access the pre-frontal cortex in the management of stressful situations.

From Enmeshment to Self-Differentiation: Dismantling Diffuse Loyalty Contracts

Individuals who enter therapy with more "benign" forms of attachment failures often describe their childhood as relatively normal. There was no real evidence of abuse or neglect, parents were described as generally loving, and there was no stress around having enough financial security to provide children with opportunities that would lead to personal and academic success. When parents deliver mixed messages around self-differentiation and/or self-worth throughout childhood, the child grows up with a type of insecure attachment that is often difficult to pinpoint. However, beneath the surface, these family environments were often laced with stories of underlying ten-sion, where anxiety or depression on the part of a parent often erupted in negative comments or accusations directed toward a child or family member that had to be witnessed and/or endured with little opportunity for ques-tioning or reparation. An unspoken stance was often created that telegraphed the need to protect the fragile family member. With these forms of loyalty contracts slights or accusations are dismissed as unimportant because verbally confronting hurtful or devaluing messages was forbidden. These family environments typically are enmeshed, where declarations of autonomy and separateness are seen as a form of betrayal.

These tenuous parental attachment styles can be easily fractured, and children quickly learn to adjust and accommodate the parent's fragility. Margaret Crastnopol (2015) refers to these situations or ruptures as micro-traumatic injurious moments that occur in relationships that are otherwise felt to be valuable, and as such there is a tendency to ignore the injury so as not to disrupt the relational connection. Yet, the impact of these injuries will accumulate over time resulting in a "psychic bruising" that leaves these individuals unable to adequately defend themselves. Crastnopol states, "Micro-traumatic experience is by definition something that is under-played, and as such, its impact remains unarticulated, dissociated, or suppressed. Because one hasn't seen the cuff coming or registered its full impact, one hasn't defended oneself adequately. One hasn't taken either the reparative or protective steps that might ease the injury in its aftermath or guard against reoccurrences. So, the damage mounts, and the result is a skewing in one's sense of goodness, efficacy, or cohesion" (p. 3).

The experience of repeated momentary fractures in communication with a parent clearly leaves the child in a state of increased vulnerability. Mitchell & Aron, 1999; Stolorow & Atwood, 1992; and Stern, 2010, remind us that a person's sense of personal cohesion, goodness, and efficacy is conveyed intersubjectively, through the verbal and non-verbal conveyance of the interpersonal, interactive matrix. It is the parent's job to help with the intersubjective repair when ruptures occur, using language to help sort through the confusion and to give the child verbal reassurance. If children are left alone with this confusion, unable to process the ruptures of repeated interpersonal interactions with a parent, these children are then left with an underlying anxiety, ill-prepared to communicate, believing that it is impossible to make sense of an unreliable, often contradictory world. They often grow up with diffuse feelings of guilt, assume a sense of over-responsibility for others, and tend to downplay the experience of being on the receiving end of slights or disappointments from others.

In comparison to individuals with more severe attachment injuries where trauma and/or neglect were pervasive, these patients are often described as the wounded-well. However, it is important not to minimize the cumulative effect that parental mixed messages, competitive pressure, or verbal slights have on the psyche. They are a form of micro-aggression that grinds the individual into a state of submission while simultaneously creating a defensive posture of over-compensation to prove self-worth. Bottom line, these individuals are left without the tools of verbal self-defense to challenge unfair behavior. Nor have they been given permission to believe that they have a right to self-protection. Acquiescence to the will of the parent creates the path of least resistance and greatest safety. Thus, a sense of malaise coupled with underlying feelings of anxiety remain just beneath the surface.

Client Example

In Chapter Two you were introduced to a young woman, a software engineer in her thirties, who had a mother who gave her mixed messages around choosing a life that was different than the one her mother chose, which was a path of self-sacrifice and loyalty to family. Throughout her childhood and young adulthood, the patient continually felt as if her mother put her in a double bind that could be summarized as, "*I want you to have the career I never was able to have. But I don't want you to have more than I was allowed to have in my life because you owe me for my sacrifice.*" The patient would often suffer from mother's withdrawal or angry accusations if she disobeyed or made a misstep. The thought of speaking up, or later in adulthood setting limits with mother filled the patient with extreme anxiety, sometimes to the point of losing her words. As a result of this insecure attachment pattern, one that was filled with mixed messages of narcissistic longings and punitive retaliation, left the patient assuming the role of family mediator and self-sufficient over-achiever. She felt guilty and tried to downplay her feelings of frustration over the way her mother refused to take responsibility for her own anxiety. She also minimized the toll that her role as family mediator took on her, stating that she could handle it and had nothing to complain about. She often would state that she was just grateful that her family afforded her as many opportunities in life as she had been given.

During the course of therapy time was spent focusing on the unfair loyalty contract. It took many months for her to acknowledge how claustrophobic her mother's hovering sometimes felt. She recalled an incident in elementary school where she had finished a school science project, went to bed, and woke up to find that her mother had completely redone the whole project. She later confessed that she felt like a fraud winning the science competition, and her mother's pride in her award left her feeling both betrayed and illegitimate. The patient confessed that she had never shared that story with anyone up to this point in her life because it filled her with so much shame. When asked what it felt like to share the story now, she reported that once she had shared the secret, she could feel herself becoming angry rather than ashamed.

As the treatment progressed, the thought of approaching her mother and confronting her verbally continued to leave her in a state of panic to the point that she would momentarily dissociate in the treatment hour. However, as the patient became more consciously aware of her mother's inability to contain her own anxiety as well as mother's inability to process disappointments in life, the patient gradually was able to separate her own anxiety from her mother's demands that the patient make her mother feel better. It was at this point that she was able to acknowledge her anger more directly to the therapist, realizing the unfairness of her childhood despite growing up in an environment of privilege. This enabled her to shift her loyalty contract within the family to a more individuated position. No longer did she come to her father's rescue, and she stopped being a peacemaker in family disputes.

In time, when the patient had interactions with her mother, she was simply able listen to her complaints without feeling the pressure to offer advice or come to the rescue. She also began to verbally challenge mother's negative assumptions and/or mixed messages. First steps in this area required pushing through her visceral, reflexive fear that her mother would sever the relationship permanently, that somehow the patient would cross a line that would create permanent damage. She tested the waters by pointing out the differing expectations that were placed on her and her brother. She wondered aloud with her mother why one set of rules applied to her an another to her brother. Although mother became defensive and accused her of misinterpreting her actions, they were able to weather this challenge without a relational rupture. Gradually, she was able to set firmer limits around parenting advice, family vacations, and finances. The patient felt that it was important to free herself from financial indebtedness to her mother, thus enabling her to experience less of a double bind.

Two years into the therapeutic process, the patient reported that her parents had decided to sell their home in Delaware and move to their daughter's hometown to be closer to grandchildren. When asked if she was concerned about the proximity, the patient responded by saying that she wasn't. Her parents were currently visiting for the past two weeks, and the patient stated that this was a good practice round for testing how well she could maintain firm boundaries. She recounted the following as she reflected on their visit:

"You would be proud of me. This time, I didn't let my mother's moods get to me. What a difference compared to last year. My dad was peach and played with the kids. Mom didn't interact with her grandchildren that much but took it upon herself to clean and cook. This time I didn't get into a struggle with her over her obsessive cleaning. Then, one morning the baby woke up at 5:30 crying. We're letting her stay in her room when she wakes up to try to self-soothe for a while, and generally she settles right down. I had mentioned that to my mother earlier. But this morning my mother stormed into our room saying – 'Aren't you going to do anything? What kind of mother are you?' I told her I had things under control and reminded her that Jessie would settle down.

She started getting more upset and told me that I was selfish and inconsiderate, and why wouldn't I just listen to her. She said she's had plenty of parenting experience too. Then she stormed off, went back into the guest bedroom, and slammed the door. I remember thinking, 'I'm dealing with a toddler right now, not an adult.' I wasn't upset and didn't feel any need to follow her and try to apologize or make her calm down. And what was amazing is that an hour later she came down for breakfast and didn't refer to the incident again. She behaved as if the outburst never happened.

The other thing that I became aware of is how my mother still uses money to try to keep control. It was my birthday last week, and my parents generally give all of us fairly large checks. She gave a substantial check to my brother two months ago. But she didn't give me one this year, only a card. Talk about a message! It's as if she's saying, 'If I'm not able to control you with the strings attached with the business loan I gave you, then I'll withhold from you by not giving you anything.' It hurts to realize this, of course. But I also realize this is her stuff not mine. In the past I would have been racked with anxiety, wondering what I had done to cause her to be so upset with me. I know I didn't do anything wrong. You know, it does makes me angry because I feel I've made so much progress, and she's made none. Or the progress she's made is because of me setting limits. She hasn't changed and probably never will. At least I can be my own person, and now I'm unscathed by the way she deals with things. (Pause) So, that's a long-winded answer saying why I'll be ok having them move closer."

I refer to this case study again in this chapter to illustrate the progress that can be made regarding insight and self-reflective capacities when clients with less severe attachment injuries are given the opportunity to work through unfair loyalty contracts that are filled with ongoing micro-traumatic exchanges between a parent and a child. Because this patient's father had a pattern of conflict avoidance when it came to managing his wife's anxiety and angry outbursts, it fell upon the patient to try to make peace and cater to mother's wishes. This created an unfair psychic burden on her that continued well into adulthood. Because the micro-traumatic exchanges within the early childhood dynamics were underplayed, the patient entered treatment at a loss as to why she was suffering from anxiety and depression. As Crastnopol (2015) points out, clearly her sense of goodness, efficacy, and self-cohesion had suffered as a result of this over-accommodating style. When this patient entered therapy, she demonstrated an anxious, overly accommodating attachment style, where she avoided conflict and tried to please others often at the expense of her own exhaustion.

In the beginning phase of treatment, this client was at a loss for words in terms of trying to identify the hostility and control that was imbedded in her mother's generosity with money and hovering attention. Hovering attention is often confused with love, and it took some time for the patient to begin to be able to articulate the mixed messages her mother often presented, such as, "You dedicate so much of yourself to your work, but I'm

*worried that you're letting yourself go. You look so tired and haggard these days."
Or "I know that your business is important to you, but you would think you would
find time to prioritize family." Or "I can't tell your father anything. He never takes
me seriously. You're the only person in this family I can confide in."*

Initially, these statements sent this patient into anxiety and confusion.
However, it was through moment-to-moment tracking of each of
mother's comments that the patient was able to see the hostility or
devaluing that was conveyed within her mother's concern. Gradually,
the patient began to question the mixed messages and asked for clarification as to what her mother meant or what she was really concerned
would happen. As she was able to verbally ask for clarification, the
patient was then able to notice how quickly her mother would respond
with defensiveness. Either mother would deny that she had said something, or she would retaliate through angry withdrawal. It was at this
point that the patient was able to grasp the extent of her mother's
fragility. She also was able to see how her mother's refusal to acknowledge her own weakness, her refusal to take medication or seek
therapeutic help for her anxiety was a decision she continued to make.
She saw the vicious cycle and the part she had been asked to play, and
this was what eventually enabled the patient to self-differentiate and
begin to set better limits, both with mother and her co-workers. The
patient's above comments and observations are a reflection of this shift,
marking the clarity that comes when feelings can be identified, affirmed,
and put into words.

Summary

Moment-to-moment tracking is at the heart of therapeutic inquiry.
Whether this technique is used in the sequential tracking of triggering
events, or it is used to mirror, reflect, or reframe parts of the patient's
beliefs, assumptions, or feeling states, the result is that patients have the
experience of being seen and heard more fully. Moment-to-moment
tracking is how the therapist slows the process down to gain further
clarification or to help move the client into a pace of interaction where
the co-regulation of affective resonance can occur. When used properly, moment-to-moment tracking is a method of crafting language
to connect right-brain-to-right-brain with patients in a way that allows
the therapist's words and reflective comments to begin to establish an
organizing structure that allows for the construction of verbal-reflective
meaning.

One of the challenges of talk therapy is learning how to hold unarticulated aspects of our clients' inner world in a way that makes the patient feel a sense of connection rather than isolation. Mirroring and naming
the felt sense of the interactive experience of underdeveloped parts of the
psyche and reflecting them back to clients is a way of using language to help

crystalize the essence of their internal experience without overwhelming them. The capacity to articulate what is being felt and observed within the therapist-client interaction enables the client to be seen, creating a state of emotional attunement, mutual influence, and affective mutuality.

Without that mirroring reflection, without the sense of being seen or recognized, the only vehicle of communication the client has to express his or her internal world is some form of enactment. As Donnel Stern (2019) states, there is a difference between words and wordlessness, what is seen as public and what is kept in private. That which cannot be expressed in words creates a pressure or a compulsion to act out. Conversely, if something can be expressed in words, the psychic pressure to act out those dimensions of unformulated experience greatly diminishes. To a similar degree, the parts of the self that are hidden or held in private often contains elements of shame and/or a sense of isolation. Bringing what is hidden or dissociated into the holding therapeutic environment in the present moment creates psychic repair through relational connection. Moment-to-moment-tracking allows the therapist to maintain attention in the unfolding present, thereby increasing the opportunity of noticing what is non-verbally expressed or hidden from view and bringing it into conscious awareness. Here is how differentiation of the self develops alongside a growing capacity for mutuality or mutual recognition in adult relationships.

References

Benjamin, J. (2018). *Beyond doer and done to: Recognition theory, intersubjectivity and the third*. Routledge.

Benjamin, J. (1988). *Bonds of love: Psychoanalysis, feminism, and the problem of domination*. Guilford Press.

Bromberg, P. (2006). *Awakening the dreamer: Clinical journeys*. Analytic Press.

Crastnopol, M. (2015).*Micro-trauma. A psychoanalytic understanding of cumulative psychic injury*. Routledge.

Danielian, J., & Gianotti, P. (2012). *Listening with purpose: Entry points into shame and narcissistic vulnerability*. Routldge.

DeRosis, L. (1974). The invented self: Karen Horney's theory applied to psychoanalysis in groups. *The American Journal of Psychoanalysis, 34*, 109–121.

Lichtenberg, J. (2001). Motivational systems and model scene with special reference to bodily experience. *Psychoanalytic Inquiry, 21*, 430–447.

Mitchell, S. A., & Aron, L. (Eds.) (1999). *Relational psychoanalysis: The emergence of a tradition*. The Analytic Press.

Stern, D. B. (2010). *Partners in thought: Working with unformulated experience, dissociation, and enactment*. Routledge.

Stern, D.B. (2019). *The infinity of the unsaid: Unformulated experience, language, and the nonverbal*. New York: Routledge.

Stolorow, R. D., & Atwood, G. E. (1992). *Contexts of being: The intersubjective foundations of psychological life*. The Analytic Press.

Sullivan, H. S. (1953). *The interpersonal theory of psychiatry.* W. W. Norton & Company, Inc.

Uddin, L. Q., Lacoboni, M., Lange, C., & Keenan, J. P. (2007). The self and social cognition: The role of cortical midline structures and mirror neurons. *Trends in Cognitive Science, 11*(4), 137–184.

Wachtel, P. (2011). *Therapeutic communication: Knowing what to say when.* The Guilford Press.

Winnicott, D. W. (1965). *The maturational processes and the facilitating environment: Studies in the theory of emotional development.* Hogarth Press and the Institute of Psychoanalysis.

6 Speaking to the Splits: Understanding the Continuum of Dissociative Process

Introduction

Neuroscientific evidence and infant research are reshaping our understanding of what it means to be in relationship with our clients. Research findings show that early traumatic experiences between the child and caregiver leave a permanent residue of damage. When these early needs for relational connection go unmet, the child perceives intense fear, helplessness, and imminent danger. Without caring intervention and repair by the caretaker, trauma is experienced. In situations of trauma, the only coping mechanism available to a child is the unconscious and physically driven capacity to dissociate early procedural memory from declarative memory. This in turn creates segregated systems of attachment, and segregated experiences of self. These segregated self-states co-exist within the personality that continue into adulthood, each split off from the other.

The effect of trauma on consciousness results in the disruption of a person's sense of continuity by retarding the linking of self-states in the course of development. People who have suffered more interruption of state linkage have more difficulty understanding their emotions and tend to feel buffeted by circumstances. Therefore, they are more like to rely on the dissociation of self-states as a means of navigating the world (Howell, 2005, p. 170). Because the splitting of self-states produces greater psychic disorganization and thus, greater challenges to therapeutic practice, this chapter is geared to helping practitioners identify and work with patients who exhibit thought processes and affective arousal states that fall within the spectrum of dissociative process.

Allan Schore (2012) encourages us to consider that "principles of early emotional development must be incorporated into an overarching model of dissociation" (p. 263). He identifies critical aspects of emotional development that lead to dissociative process as deriving from caregivers who are inaccessible, inconsistent, and respond to their infant's expressions of distress inappropriately and rejectingly. These parents either display extreme levels of stimulation/arousal, such as in abuse, or they exhibit very low responses, such as in neglect. Because there is no

DOI: 10.4324/9781003120278-7

opportunity for interactive repair, the infant's intense negative states last for long periods of time, creating a prolonged state of hyperarousal. Frequently, a secondary reaction to these repeated states of "frantic distress' results in a hypo-aroused state of dissociation, where "the child disengages from stimuli in the external world and attends to an 'internal' world" (p. 266). Schore reports that these infants are often observed as staring off into space with a glazed look and cites Kestenberg's (1985) description where he refers to "dead spots in the infant's subjective experience" (p. 266). These dead spots or this withdrawal from the external world are what we now understand as dissociative process.

Advances in neuroscience have helped us confirm that dissociation is a neurologically based involuntary reflex. When a vulnerable infant or young child is overly stimulated and fails to receive attuned affect regulation from a parent figure, the self freezes in reflexive self-protection. Schore explains that there is a loss of vertical connectivity between cortical and subcortical areas of the right hemisphere of the brain (2012, p. 277). However, this also creates a disconnect between left brain and right brain modes of organizing experience. Therefore, verbal thought processes also become compromised, even though dissociation is a right brain phenomenon. Based on the above research, therapeutic approaches aimed at the repair of early relational damage must be adapted to include ways of communicating with the patient's implicit memory system.

We are currently witnessing a gradual shift in psychodynamic approaches in the use of language as a communication tool, moving from an over-reliance on left-brain interpretations that resonate with patients' explicit memory processes to finding ways to connect with patients right-brain-to-right-brain. This shift in thinking involves directing our attention to sensorimotor components of our clients' experience in ways that attend to shifts in body language, eye contact, speech, while also observing increases in agitation, or postures that reflect emotional shut-down. It is the therapist's job to give language to these sensory-motor observations (enactments), thus bringing them into consciousness through the process of relational interaction.

Therefore, when working with patients, new modes of treatment must include a combination of perspectives that attend to:

- defense structures, albeit protective, that are based on learned attachment patterns and the enactments that become a part of self-identity and relational experience,
- an understanding of neurological hardwiring and the traumatic damage that ensues due to failures of attunement, and
- an arousal system that is largely reflexive and outside of conscious awareness.

This chapter will address each of these aspects represented within the continuum of splitting and dissociative process. Client examples will be provided to help the practitioner become more adept at recognizing and "speaking to the splits." These examples will range from mild, or micro-dissociative episodes (Crastnopol, 2015) that are frequently witnessed in the treatment hour, to more pervasive splits as found in borderline personality organization. Finally, we will examine how to recognize split off parts of the self that represent the unformulated, unarticulated or "not-me" experiences that are expressed through enactments within the treatment relationship.

The work from the Boston Change Process Study Group (2010) reminds us that enactments become the vehicle by which our patients bring dissociated material into the treatment. It is the therapist's job to give language to these unconscious enactments thus bringing them into consciousness through the process of relational interaction. This chapter will focus on how to introduce language into the relational exchange in ways that mirror and hold our patients' inner experience without overwhelming, flooding, or shaming them.

Splitting and Dissociation

Throughout the literature the terms splitting and dissociation are often used interchangeably and represent a range of meanings depending on one's theoretical frame of reference. Splitting is often considered a form of dissociative process, although historically it has had a more limited meaning, one that emphasizes the contradictory aspects of experience. As a defense mechanism, splitting divides experience into good and bad, all or nothing. When either of these two poles are emotionally triggered, one can witness an oscillation of reactivity ranging from intense rage often coupled with behavioral retaliation vs. an over-idealizing passivity and/or helplessness. Splitting is often seen in underdeveloped personalities, such as borderline or narcissistic personality disorders, where individuals actually split a single entity into two opposing realities. Because of this, they cannot integrate disparate parts of themselves or others into a cohesive whole.

Elizabeth Howell (2005) understands splitting as a posttraumatic response stemming from insecure or disorganized attachment patterns. She states, "What we call "splitting" involves a reenactment of posttraumatic dominant-submissive relational patterns. In this process, a particular organization of alternating dissociated helpless/victim and abusive/rageful self-states develops on the axis of relational trauma. These self-states reflect the impact of relational trauma on defenses, on neurological hardwiring, and on arousal systems" (p. 163).

Self-states are either integrated and fluid as is evidenced in heathy populations or they are split apart due to parental inconsistency that creates an insecure attachment. Otto Kernberg (1975) explained, the motivation for splitting is to protect the good or tender aspects of the parental relationship from being overwhelmed by the terrifying aspects of the bad. This splitting apart mechanism, referred to by self-psychologists as vertical splitting, is defined by Arnold Goldberg (1999) as a condition that originates in childhood stemming from a parent's inability to form or maintain an integrated image of the child that results in a vertical split within the child which functions as a defense against anxiety and depression (p. 31). Patricia DeYoung (2015) describes vertical splitting as "a kind of affect regulation," a right-brain response to certain specific negative emotions. She states, "The disintegration that happens in that moment is linked with specific 'dangerous' self-states (such as anger, pride, need, or sexual feeling) and the dissociation that happens sequesters just in that self-state" (p. 70). In other words, splitting serves the function of providing relief to the child from feeling unbearable emotional pain due to the feared loss of parental connection or disapproval.

The definition of dissociation encompasses a broader scope, one that captures a multitude of states, ranging from healthy to maladaptive means of compartmentalizing experience. From a clinical standpoint, dissociation refers to the separation of mental and experiential contents that would normally be connected. James Chu (1998) refers to dissociation as "a disruption of the normal integration of experience." Phillip Bromberg (1998) explains that, "The essence of dissociation is that the mind is disconnected from the psyche-soma to protect one's illusion of unitary selfhood from the potential threat of traumatically impinging experience it cannot process cognitively" (p. 232). Frank Putnam (1989) simply states that, "Dissociation represents a failure of integration of ideas, information, affects, and experience" (p. 19).

As our theoretical understanding has evolved, Donnel Stern (2010) explains that dissociation is not necessarily a defense against thoughts, feelings, or memories, but it is a defense against a *state of identity*. Depending upon the degree of trauma that was suffered, the consequent extent of dissociative defense structures will vary enormously. When trauma is so severe that it is terrifying, vicious, or abject, the state of vulnerability experienced by the child can be catastrophic, provoking massive affective dysregulation or psychotic decompensation (p. 120). In these situations, parts of the person's identity must remain unknown, split off from other self-states because the fear of psychic annihilation is so terrifying that it had to be disavowed, remaining "not known." If one were to consciously acknowledge these aspects of experience, it would mean that life would not be bearable. Stern is clear to point out that the etiology of dissociation isn't always linked to overt abuse. The cause can be any "unbearable experience" in the parent-child relationship that the self cannot own.

Research conducted by Lyons-Ruth et al. (2006) supports Stern's understanding of the damage that is created by early childhood traumatic experiences. Her findings show that children of unresponsive caretakers are more likely to engage in dissociative behaviors, and disorganized patterns of infant attachment are potential precursors to dissociation later in life.

Dissociative self-states are activated by extreme affective arousal that overwhelm the individual's physiological capacity to process stimulation. Self-states could not be integrated with the rest of experience, often as a result of traumatizing and/or neglectful environments. For example, states of terror do not get linked with other states of mind.

The Function of Dissociative Process

If one is to provide effective trauma treatment, it is important to first understand the range of functions that encompass dissociative process. Separating or compartmentalizing aspects of reality can reflect healthy, positive capacities as well as more primitively driven, limiting defense responses. It is important to understand the range of these responses, as we all exhibit degrees of compartmentalization both healthy and defensively based.

Fischer and Ayoub (1994) point out that affective splitting is a natural developmental state as children acquire skills in structuring their experience. They explain that the mind is "naturally fractionated," and in the course of development children acquire progressively more complex skills for evaluating their environment and processing reality. Over time individuals will also develop biases based on how they evaluate their emotional reactions as they impact personal goals and concerns. "Because of the pervasiveness of fractionation, people often do not even recognize elements that go together in the world. When we encounter a task that is complex or confusing for us, we simplify it by dropping out components or splitting it into separate tasks" (p. 154). Their findings confirm that splitting and dissociation occur within the normal developmental trajectory; however, in situations of childhood abuse or neglect, the integration of these separate, contextually segregated strand of meaningful experience will be impeded (Fischer & Ayoub, 1994; Putnam, 1997). Thus, it is important to understand the use of dissociation and splitting as a way of organizing experience that falls on a continuum ranging from healthy to defensive means of organizing reality.

In 1986 Eve Carlson and Frank Putnam created the "Dissociative Experiences Scale," a clinical tool that provided a means of quantifying the range of dissociative experience. Putnam (1997) described three dissociation-related functions as follows:

a. to divide attention into two or more streams of consciousness,
b. to compartmentalize information and/or affect, and
c. to alter one's identity and create distance from oneself.

Let us examine each of these in more detail. The first of Putnam's dissociative functions, the ability to *divide attention into two or more streams of consciousness,* is what I would call a healthy form of dissociation. Examples of this are daydreaming, multi-tasking, or getting lost in thought to the point that you miss your exit on a highway. Often referred to as multiplicity of mind, which is something none of us could do without, we can think of normal dissociative process as a collection of multiple self-states, corresponding to role and context that shift continuously in our lives. In a very basic sense, normal dissociation encompasses the ability to: focus our attention, separate figure from ground, and engage in deep states of concentration. Csikszentmihalyi (2008) refers to healthy dissociation as a "flow experience" where flow is described as a state of mind that is harmoniously ordered to the point that one can get lost in a pleasurable activity, such as art, music, yoga, a good book, sports, or any creative pursuit that stretches the mind to higher challenges (p. 6).

The second form of dissociation is *the ability to compartmentalize information and affect.* Janina Fisher (2021) describes this experience as "transient amnestic or depersonalization responses that give us distance from overwhelming events that allow us to be 'there' but 'not there.' Compartmentalization allows us to live with otherwise irreconcilable conflicts or avoid cognitive dissonance" (p. 2). Jack Danielian and I (2012) refer to this as a permeable state of knowing and not knowing, where disparate self-states are in conflict to the point that varying degrees of compartmentalization can occur. Examples of this type of conflictual knowing and not knowing range from buying bottled water for its convenience even though we know plastics are polluting our environment, to continuing to maintain an idealized loyalty contract with a parent or partner who is abusive, to having an affair and telling yourself your actions won't hurt your partner. Although a form of compartmentalization happens in healthy dissociation, the process is not triggered by painful affect, cognitive dissonance, or an irreconcilable conflict.

The third type of dissociation is described as the *altering of identity and creating distance from the self.* This form of dissociative process is entirely defensively driven, inhibiting the psychic integration of various self-states. Phenomena such as depersonalization, derealization, psychic numbing, experiencing oneself as floating above one's body, going into fugue states, or experiencing the loss of time cover a spectrum of examples of this type of distancing from the self. Professional actors and public speakers represent a less fractured state of altering one's identity. Here is where a relatively shy or introverted person can assume the role of a bold or angry individual by accessing a self-state considered outside of one's normal identity. However, with more defensively driven states where traumatically induced dissociation functions to alter identity, individual experience a sense of discomfort, confusion, or disorganization. Depending on the severity of early attachment failures, traumatic dissociative process involves a fracturing of the self or a neuro-physiological shutting down in order to preserve homeostasis.

Phillip Bromberg (1998) states that psychological self-continuity plays a central role in all human life. Bromberg (2006) clarifies that dissociative process falls on a continuum. He explains that although the adaptive function of dissociation in individuals with trauma histories help maintain a sense of self-continuity and self-organization, there is also a cost. These individuals have a decreased capacity to tolerate internal conflict, and they show a diminished capacity for intersubjectivity and mentalization due to experiences that were so overwhelming or occurred too early in life that they weren't encoded in language or organized symbolically.

Allan Schore (2012) refers to traumatic dissociation as a state where implicit right-brain functioning loses its synaptic activity to the point that it fails to recognize and process external stimuli, where the individual is unable to integrate external stimuli with internal emotional experience. Due to chaotic ruptures of regulation or the parent's inability to co-regulate and soothe affective arousal in early childhood, both subjectivity and intersubjectivity collapse within the awareness of the child (p. 160). These repeated ruptures fall outside of explicit memory or conscious self-awareness; however, the pain and damage are internalized and can be recognized through defensive enactments that fluctuate between attempts to keep feelings of shame at bay by enacting behavioral over-compensation vs. the break-through of feelings of self-loathing and/or despair that results in dissociative shut-down. Schore states that individuals with severe attachment failures often report an inability to sustain an inner sense of aliveness (p. 126). Thus, the shutting down of painful relational ruptures take their toll on a person's sense of self-congruence.

Splitting, Dissociation and the Four Quadrant Model: Understanding Self-States Through the Lens of Part-Whole Analysis

One way to conceptualize splitting and dissociative process is to think about the psyche as being organized into relatively integrated or disconnected self-states. Steven Kuchuck (2021) defines self-states as "separate, individual units of being within the psyche" (p. 81). Each of these states are comprised of thoughts, beliefs, emotions, memories, behaviors, and values that either result in an overall state of coherence or states that may become more or less dissociated from one another. Kuchuck reminds us that relationally based theoretical models view the self not as "a singular entity but rather a non-linear, shifting collection of separate self-states moving in and out of dissociation/consciousness and psychic dominance while in a dialectic with the adaptive illusion of a singular self (p. 82)."

Donnel Stern (2010) explains that the various harmonious and/or conflicting purposes within the personality are experienced as "parts" of us, as "states" of our selves. When there is a history of trauma, "the child cannot bear to experience simultaneously states that were created in the presence of safety and others created during the appearance of a dangerous, traumatic person... ("angry-father" for example)" (p. 85). It is as if the child must protect the positive experience of safety by removing the dangerous situation and/or terrifying feeling states from consciousness. Later in adulthood, Stern states that these traumatic memories or self-states remain unknown consciously although they can be witnessed through repeated behavioral enactments, while the individual "lives" his or her own life inside the more bearable and consciously integrated self-states.

Think of the Four Quadrant Model as a picture of various self-states with various parts of the self in fluid, integrated connection or as self-states split off from one another. The connections, disconnections, and interactions between these parts in relation to the whole are what comprise the realm of each individual's subjective experience. In other words, the Four Quadrant structure is a picture of personality organization that reflects the outcome of attachment failures where the child/now adult continues to make attempts to correct or compensate for early failures or losses.

If we draw from Fischer and Ayoub's description of fractionation as a means of understanding defensive splitting/dissociation, where the reduction of emotional complexity helps maintain psychic coherence, we can see how early attachment failures become internalized self-states, either known, partially known, or unformulated.

Self-states manifest as patterns or biases (Character Solutions) that reduce aspects of reality and amplify others. The Four Quadrants show the relationship between self-states that are to some degree fractionated or unformulated due to unbearable feelings of terror, shame, or lack of acceptance. Each quadrant represents "a part" of the organizational landscape consisting of beliefs about self-worth, relational expectations, and behavioral strategies for how one navigates the world. The Four Quadrant Model is included below for your further reference.

Viewing each of the quadrants as self-states, Quadrants Two and Four can be understood as parts of the self that are to some degree split off from consciously accepted hopes, wishes, and dreams for the self in relationship. In a sense the feelings generated from Quadrants Two and Four create a cognitive dissonance within the personality, challenging self-esteem, and fantasied self-attributions. Because the Four Quadrant Model is a picture of defensively based strategies of over-compensation, disconnection between *any* of the four quadrants represents a window into understanding the damage that is created when a vulnerable child is not met with safety, consistency, mutuality, or support. The Four Quadrant Model, unlike the Healthy Self-Actualizing Model, represents a hoped-for idealized version of the self that was manufactured through fantasy and imagination. The parts of the self that are not represented within the fantasied longings or personal narrative then become split off and remain disavowed or unknown, only to be made manifest in the treatment hour through reported enactments in the outside world and within the therapeutic relationship.

Karen Horney (1950) identified the relationship between two powerful self-states, pointing out how a person's omnipotent idealized images of the

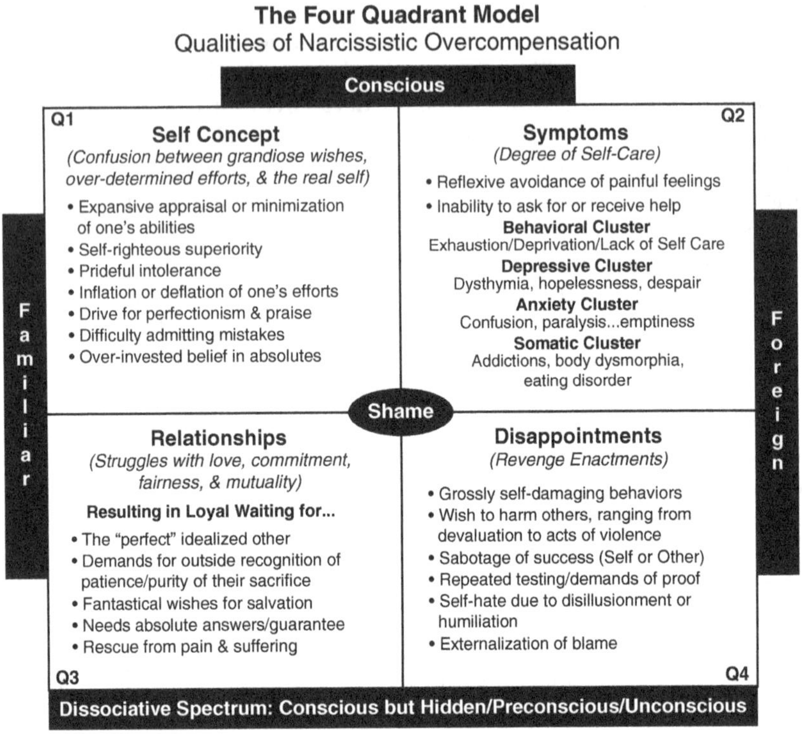
The Four Quadrant Model
Qualities of Narcissistic Overcompensation
Conscious
Q1
Self Concept
(Confusion between grandiose wishes, over-determined efforts, & the real self)
• Expansive appraisal or minimization of one's abilities
• Self-righteous superiority
• Prideful intolerance
• Inflation or deflation of one's efforts
• Drive for perfectionism & praise
• Difficulty admitting mistakes
• Over-invested belief in absolutes
Q2
Symptoms
(Degree of Self-Care)
• Reflexive avoidance of painful feelings
• Inability to ask for or receive help
Behavioral Cluster
Exhaustion/Deprivation/Lack of Self Care
Depressive Cluster
Dysthymia, hopelessness, despair
Anxiety Cluster
Confusion, paralysis...emptiness
Somatic Cluster
Addictions, body dysmorphia, eating disorder
Familiar
Foreign
Shame
Relationships
(Struggles with love, commitment, fairness, & mutuality)
Resulting in Loyal Waiting for...
• The "perfect" idealized other
• Demands for outside recognition of patience/purity of their sacrifice
• Fantastical wishes for salvation
• Needs absolute answers/guarantee
• Rescue from pain & suffering
Q3
Disappointments
(Revenge Enactments)
• Grossly self-damaging behaviors
• Wish to harm others, ranging from devaluation to acts of violence
• Sabotage of success (Self or Other)
• Repeated testing/demands of proof
• Self-hate due to disillusionment or humiliation
• Externalization of blame
Q4
Dissociative Spectrum: Conscious but Hidden/Preconscious/Unconscious

Figure 6.1 The Four Quadrant Model.

self can co-exist in a non-linear relationship with (corrosive) images of self-hate. Together, she explains, they fuel in the patient a systemic sense of false pride. "False pride and its' accompanying 'systemic shame' are critical factors in the damaging splits that maintain a tightly homeostatic systemic balance" (Danielian & Gianotti, 2012). Depending upon the degree of defensive over-compensation, the degree of dissociative splitting will be more or less pervasive in an attempt to create a homeostatic balance and avoid psychic fragmentation. Patricia DeYoung (2021) points out that dissociation can often create a barrier between different self-states. For example, a client may feel confident and optimistic in one self-state, and the next day may feel a sense of deep despair, without having any memory of one state while in the other. Whereas people who experience less severe levels of dissociation don't decompensate so dramatically when dysregulation strikes, and they are able to recover and reconnect with self and others more easily.

The degree to which these self-states are integrated or split apart determines the degree of psychic stability and/or fragility. Therapists often unwittingly fall victim to colluding with patients around maintaining the split off parts of the psyche, whether they fail to recognize or minimize a split, or they normalize grandiose defenses that function to hide feelings of shame. This is why the Four Quadrant Model and Healthy Self-Actualizing Model were designed – to help stretch our ability to see more and more of the parts that represent the complexity of the psyche, both healthy and pathological. Attending to the dialectic tension between and within these self-systems allows us to better identify the connection or disconnection that comprises the individual's psychic organization. Gradually, more and more parts of the patient's psyche will be revealed as the treatment progresses. Understanding the inter-relationship between the quadrants helps us spot parts of the psyche that may be hidden or unknown to the client.

How to Recognize Splitting within the Clinical Hour

It takes a little practice to recognize when signs of splitting are revealed within the clinical hour. Often when I review process recordings with student trainees, I will ask, "Did you see how this statement represents a split?" Many times, the response is a puzzled, "No." Splitting can be explained in the most simplistic sense as attending to *a part of something* and treating it as if it *the whole of something*. Unfortunately, this way of organizing reality is becoming more of the norm. Much of our political discourse and media coverage is based on oversimplification or treating a part of something as if it were the whole. As a result, oversimplified explanations have been normalized to the point that many people fail to register when a split is occurring. Alternatively, therapists also report that they are at a loss as to how to address splitting in a helpful way without increasing defensiveness, thus running the risk of shaming the patient or creating a breach in the alliance.

Splitting can manifest in a number of ways depending on the severity of the fracture. When it comes to increasing one's ability to recognize a split off part, you can begin by paying attention to patterns that point to a lack of integration between thoughts, beliefs, or actions. Types of splitting can be identified by:

- Splitting the affective component from the intellectual recall of an event or memory.
- Splitting two affectively charged states – good vs. bad, creating a tendency to blame out or blame in.
- Splitting mind from body, external from internal, with an overemphasis on one vs. the other.
- Ignoring or minimizing parts of the whole because they threaten/contradict current beliefs and assumption.
- Failure to accurately assess a dangerous situation often resulting in high-risk behaviors.

- Minimizing the impact of a painful event or excusing the actions of others to protect one's idealized wishes in hopes that things will be different next time.
- Exhibiting a fuzziness in thinking, tracking, sequencing.
- Exhibiting a sense of depersonalization or derealization.
- Splitting to the degree that one cannot remember one state while in the other.

Each of these examples represent a type of dissociative split that serves the purpose of homeostatic stabilization. These are reflexive responses created to; a). protect the individual from potential ruptures in attachment, or b). to reduce the likelihood of personal danger and/or feelings of shame. Although these types of fractionation were once useful for self-stabilization and affect regulation in childhood, these reflexive patterns signify split-off parts of the personality that are so threatening that they cannot be integrated into conscious narrative. When activation occurs within the session, it is more likely that we will witness a micro-dissociative episode as we track the dialogic exchange.

Below is a partial list of actual client statements that illustrate how individuals rationalize their thought processes to keep parts disconnected from other parts.

1. A patient begins to describe a humiliating event from childhood but seems disconnected from any emotion. When asked about the impact, the patient might say any number of the following statements: *I just decide not to think about it. I put it out of my mind. The past is the past. I don't let myself feel because it's a sign of weakness.*
2. A patient experiences powerful affective reactions (nightmares, sudden panic), but can't connect the emotions with any recognizable trigger and states: *"I suddenly get overwhelmed with a terrible fear, but I don't know where it is coming from."*
3. Both content and affect are split-off from awareness, but disconnected bodily symptoms are present (nausea, choking, blandness). A patient might say: *"There's nothing there. I don't know what to say. I can't breathe."*
4. The patient can connect with cognition or affect, or two opposing affective states separately, but cannot experience them together. (When one part is in awareness, the other part drops out of memory and awareness): *"Did I just say that? I don't remember saying that."*

Just as it is important to recognize when splitting occurs in the session, it is equally important to catch when the integration of split-off material is being incorporated into the whole. Here are several examples of the integration of splits. The first is an example of a person who had split his feelings of terror from his cognitive recall of past events. This is the patient's recount of what happened when the affective impact of how he was parented finally hit him.

> "*I felt very rattled and nervous after our last session. In fact, when I left to go out for a little lunch afterwards, I was still nervous and shaky. Before I started this treatment, I knew my family's narrative. I mean I knew it was bad, that my parents weren't equipped to be parents at all, and I knew that it had crippled my development. And I've had to do so much therapy to get to the point of even admitting that to myself. But, since we've begun our work together, it seems to be hitting me in a different way. I mean, I knew that my parents' limitations were real, but all this time I knew it as if it were just a story. But now I'm connecting the reality of what happened to how it affected me emotionally. That all hit me at the end of our session, right when I sat down in the restaurant. And when that happened, I couldn't stop shaking.*"

This is a clear illustration of what happens when the emotional component of a memory gradually become integrated. Often this integration is felt on a body-level, as if the body's own means of storing memory is finally offered up to the parts of the psyche that have encoded experience in declarative memory self-states. When the patient shared this story, the therapist and patient were together able to acknowledge the seriousness and importance of this event, even celebrate it as a victory. In the following weeks and months what followed this moment of affective integration was a gradual shift in other areas of his life. The patient was then able to acknowledge the numerous times he had minimized himself or his own needs in various relationships past and present. Slowly, he began to advocate for himself more directly while gaining more confidence as his depression began to lift.

A second example highlights the integration of a self-state where the patient is able to see her child self from the point of view of a more benevolent, compassionate place within her current adult self.

> "*It's so sad. It's like I'm looking at myself in a movie and I'm watching the movie as an adult right now and wanting to just jump into the screen to protect that tired teenager who essentially was living like an adult. Why did I ever think I wasn't good enough? I never got to be a kid. Damn them for not taking care of me. I couldn't stand up for myself then. I was too scared. It's all I knew. It's what they told me I had to live up to.*"

This illustration brings together two self-states, one that holds the memory of a neglected child and the other that now sees from a healthy adult vantage-point how the child-self wasn't cared for by her parent. Once the adult self-state can understand how the conditions of neglect put her child self in an impossible situation, her conscious narrative can change, and she can now begin to make different choices in life. She can hold the child self with compassion and integrate her into a more coherent, protected place within her expanded/modified narrative.

This third example illustrates how the observing self is able to stop a conversational exchange when the patient realizes that he has fallen into an old pattern.

> *"So, I was talking to him and then I realized I had brushed off his kind words. Then, I stopped. I interrupted myself and said, Wait a minute. I want to go back to what just happened a moment ago. You were trying to stay connected with me, and I brushed you off. That's my pattern, and I just wanted you to know that I noticed that I did that again."*

The power of the phrase *Wait a minute* is a way to press the pause button on automatic response patterns. It is something that as therapists we do from the beginning of treatment, and eventually, we hope that the capacity to take a reflective pause becomes internalized within our patients. As I responded to my patient, I mentioned that in taking the reflective pause to say, *wait a minute* out loud, he had actually changed his old pattern in that moment. By verbalizing what he had noticed, he called the person across from him back into connection with him. I then shared that when I reflected on our treatment, I had been saying a version of 'wait a minute' to him from the very beginning of our relationship. *"Wait a minute. I don't see you as a difficult person. I see you trying to speak your mind." "Wait a minute. I wouldn't call that defiant or selfish. How I understand your need to say no to your mother was your attempt to resist her constant hovering and need to control you." What a minute. Of course, you have a right to be angry. What your partner did in that meeting was disrespectful to the whole group. Just because no one said anything, doesn't mean your feelings weren't justified."* And on and on throughout the therapy, until my patient began to make an internal shift toward self-advocacy. He thought about this and laughed saying, *"Yeah, I was coming to you for therapy, and I really thought I was better at analyzing myself than letting you do your job."* But this is how relational patterns play themselves out between the therapist and the client. It generally takes some time before the enactments are interrupted by the pause to consider new ways of seeing and being in the world.

Speaking to the Splits

The art of verbally reflecting what we notice when we see dissociative splits or fractures unfold within the clinical hour must be done in a caring, gentle, non-judgmental fashion. In a manner of speaking, what we are attempting to do is translate patient enactments that reflect implicit, encoded memory processes and verbalize them in a way that their right brain, implicit memory system can *feel* our understanding of their experience. Because dissociative splits are primarily revealed through behavioral enactments, they largely remain unregistered within the patient's organizing schemas until they are verbally articulated by a caring other. Hearing another speak the unspoken is a powerful form of holding and being seen in relationship. Verbally connecting parts that are in conscious awareness to other dissociated parts is a way of connecting explicit/declarative memory processes with the client's implicit/emotional self-states. Speaking to the splits by verbally connecting parts to other parts provides an intermediary function that eventually promotes the formation of coherent and more expansive personal narratives.

As therapists we can learn to "speak to the splits" by *wondering about something together with our patients*. For example,

- we can wonder about how the patient came to have the reactions they have to certain behaviors, beliefs, or events.
- we can gradually begin to verbalize their unspoken or disavowed wishes and longings that are expressed through their desires and their disappointments.
- we can begin to name and normalize feelings that are considered taboo or overwhelming, thus giving permission for tender feelings of vulnerability and painful feelings of shame come to the surface.
- finally, we can gradually reflect our patients' contradictory statements back to them, holding both sides of the split so that they can *hear* the split being articulated verbally.

It is one thing to recognize a statement that might reflect dissociative splitting. It is another thing to find ways to respond that draw attention to the split that are clear, succinct, and non-shaming. Often student trainees will say, "I was aware that they were jumping from one topic to another," or "I was aware that the statement he made just contradicted what he said ten minutes ago, but I didn't know what to say next." For training purposes, it is often helpful to hear multiple examples of how a therapist *might* respond to connect two split-off parts to one another. In our consultation groups, we spend time practicing several different ways a therapist might speak to the same statement that contains split off elements.

The following section lists several actual statements from patients that reveal some degree of dissociative splitting in action. Each patient statement is followed by several therapist responses that illustrate a variety of ways to make a reflective comment that speaks to the split.

Client Example One

The first patient statement represents a split between a longing for connection/appreciation (Q3) followed by a reflexive retaliatory action when disappointed (Q4). The patient is not consciously aware that these two self-states are connected. Nor is he aware of what causes the abrupt switch from one self-state to the other. In addition, there is no awareness that his longing and the subsequent way he handles disappointment reflects a recapitulation of the patient's relationship with his father.

Pt. Statement: **"I try to give people a lot of slack. I bend over backwards being generous and kind, but then when they start taking advantage of me, I'm done. They are dead to me."**

Therapist Response Example #1: It sounds as if you're trying so hard to be generous with people, but then when you realize that your behavior isn't making them change, you cut them off pretty quickly. It's as if something gets triggered in you and then it seems as if a switch flips inside of you. Can we look at how that happens?

Therapist Response Example # 2: When you get to the point that you say "I'm done," that seems to happen almost as a reflex. Maybe we can slow things down so that I can understand more of what happens when you get disappointed or when the frustration hits you.

Therapist Response Example #3: What do you mean when you say, dead to me? Is that what your father did when he was disappointed or upset with people? Did he cut them off? I wonder if you felt dead inside when he did that to you?

Analysis

Each of the therapist's responses attend to the actual words that the patient said but connect those words or phrases with other "parts" of the patient's history that the therapist suspects may be at play. One of the key components to successfully speaking to the splits is inviting patients to slow down enough so that they can examine what might be under the surface of their automatic responses. In this patient's situation, there is no middle ground. There is no verbal processing of minor disappointments as they happen. There is just the self-state of giving and being generous (enactment of the longing) or there is the self-state of complete shut-down (enactment of the disappointment). Also, the phrase "They are dead to me," reflects painful and/or confusing affect that is under the surface, but the patient is not consciously aware of the split emotions – fear of being cut off from father and becoming dead inside, vs. anger and punishment for having his longings for connection be disappointed. Speaking to both of these emotional states can gradually bring the affect components of this pattern into conscious awareness.

Client Example Two

The second patient statement represents a split between feelings of suicidality followed by the minimization of this feeling state as being real and/or important. This is a repeated pattern for the patient, one that results in frequent emergency service calls to the local mental health center.

When asked about this by the therapist several days later, here is the patient's response.

Patient Statement: **Well, sure. I was talking about not really caring if I live or die, and I may have mentioned the word suicide. I know that kind of freaked Mary out, but I am really not suicidal now. So, I don't want anyone to get all up in arms and start talking about sending me to a hospital. It's not a big deal, and I wish people wouldn't get all reactive; it just makes everything worse. I'm fine now. And don't you start getting on my case either.**

Therapist Response Example #1: So, because you are not feeling suicidal right now, does that mean that you don't think these feelings will come up in the future? How would you want people to respond when you tell people that you don't care if you live or die?

Therapist Response Example #2: Please know that by bringing this up I'm not upset or disappointed with you right now. I'm a little confused, and I'm just trying to understand. When you say you're not suicidal now, I'm still concerned about the times when you do dip into pretty deep places of depression. When you say you're fine now, do you want me to forget about the other parts of you that are suffering? I think it's important that we try to understand both of these parts of yourself, even though you may be feeling fine at the moment.

Therapist Response Example #3: By asking you about this today, that doesn't mean that I'm ready to put you in the hospital. You know, it's ok for you to admit to me how badly you feel sometimes. I'm just trying to understand what makes you feel fine today and not fine two days ago. Those are both places inside of you that are important to talk about together. What's it like to hear me say this to you right now?

Analysis

The three possible responses from the therapist attempt to speak to both sides of the split, each in slightly different ways, but each invite the patient to reconnect with the therapist as an ally. The first response reminds the patient of both sides of the split but asks her to tell the therapist how people should respond if she is on the more frightening part of the split. This encourages the patient to imagine what it is like for other people to hear her words, but it also gives her the control over imagining how she might be able to receive help at those difficult times. The second and third responses speak to the two self-states as parts of herself that co-exist inside of her, regardless of how much she wants to push the depressed, suicidal part away in that moment. The second response offers reassurance against feelings of fear or shame for having possibly disappointed the therapist. The third response invites the patient to respond to the therapist's concern for her in the present moment, in hopes that her question will reaffirm their connection to one another. All three of these responses speak to relational connectivity in addition to addressing the split directly.

Client Example Three

The third patient statement occurred shortly after hearing that her father had been living a double life. While the father was in the hospital recovering from a heart attack, she received a letter from the father's other wife asking if she could visit him in the hospital. The patient then confronted her father only to realize that the two marriages had been going on for decades.

Patient Statement: **I mean I was in high school and working at the business full time. I barely had a normal teenage life with friends because of working and school. Now sitting here, I realize the last thing I should be thinking about was that my father might be leading a double life. But, should I have known? He was gone a lot and always said it was for business. How could I be so stupid? I just didn't look for it. But, wait, why should I have looked for anything? I was a kid. And I felt like I had to because my mom didn't. She was so naïve. And I was always so close to my dad, his favorite. Now I've lost that. Everything feels like it's ruined. Maybe I'm over-reacting. I just don't know."**

Therapist Response Example #1: I can see that you're struggling with this news. This is a huge shock, and it's normal to have so many mixed emotions and questions. But I hear you beating yourself up a little bit because you are telling yourself you should have known. You tried to take care of everything when you were a teenager. There was so much pressure. I'm wondering if you're putting pressure on yourself right now, telling yourself you should have known something that no young girl could have known. Wouldn't it be ok just to feel the shock and grief over this news without being so hard on yourself?

Therapist Response Example # 2: I know this is pretty shocking news about your father. But I hear something else that's going on inside of you. There seems to be a part of you that is beating yourself up for not knowing about this and another part of you that is starting to feel protective of that teenager that was overworked and couldn't possibly have known everything that was going on in your family at that time. It almost feels like these two parts of yourself are a little bit at war with each other. Are you aware of those two different parts of yourself?

Therapist Response Example #3: I'm wondering if you're blaming yourself because somehow not knowing would mean you were naïve like your mother. Are you ashamed of that? I know you weren't close to your mother as a teenager, and your closeness with your dad helped keep you steady. Hearing this about your father is quite a loss. I'm wondering if now you're struggling with where your loyalties should lie. It's going to take time to sort all of this out.

Analysis

Each of the therapist's responses attempt to offer comfort to the patient as she wrestles with how to process this shocking news. The first response directs the patient to examine how much pressure she is putting on herself and gives her permission to simply feel the shock and grief, rather than expecting herself to have somehow known about father's double life. The second response directs the patient's attention to the ambivalent struggle she is feeling regarding two opposing self-states. The therapist verbally notices that there is an emerging part of her that doesn't want to constantly feel pressure to know everything and do the right thing all the time. She supports this emerging self-state by wondering what it would be like for the patient to simply let herself feel compassion for the overworked, dutiful teenager that she was. The third response connects the patient's shock with her shame of being naïve like her mother, but then the therapist begins to introduce the idea of misplaced family loyalties into the conversation.

In this client example we see how old loyalty contracts have played out. This news creates an opportunity for the therapist to begin to explore the patient's assumptions about what it meant to be a dutiful daughter and her father's favorite. Hearing the news about her father creates an opening for the patient to begin wondering about family dynamics in general, whereas father's actions had remained unquestioned or unacknowledged in the past. All three of the above responses represent different ways to enter into the exploration of the old loyalty contract, allowing the patient to begin to let go of her over-determined efforts to achieve success and remain in connection.

Client Example Four

This is a case where a fifteen-year-old adolescent patient was discovered cutting herself. The cutting, which had been going on for several months, had been undetected by mother for weeks because the girl cut herself in places that were normally hidden by clothing. When the therapist explored where the underlying tension might be coming from, she noted that the patient's current living situation is evenly divided between time with mother and equal time with father. There was a previous long custody battle where mother tried to gain full custody but failed, and tension remained between mother and father. In addition, father is a former drug addict, continues to exert control over both his ex-wife and daughter, and has a history of being very secretive. Recently, father has asked his daughter not to talk to her mother about what goes on when she spends time with dad.

Patient Statement: **There's nothing wrong with me. I'm fine. I don't know what the big deal is about cutting. I only did it once or twice. I'm fine.**

Therapist Response Example #1: I believe that a part of you may tell yourself that you're just fine. And I know that you don't want people to worry about you. But there is another part of you, the part of you that is cutting yourself, that may actually be wanting people know that you're not fine.

Therapist Response Example #2: I know that a part of you is trying to tell me that you're just fine. But I'm wondering what the part of you that is cutting yourself is trying to let people know? If those cuts could speak, what would they say?

Therapist Response Example #3: Cutting yourself doesn't mean that you're just fine. I want you to know that I take it seriously. That's because I value your life and I'm here to help you. You don't have to be embarrassed or minimize this. You know, when I express my concern, it doesn't mean that I'm judging you. I'm here to try to understand, to listen to whatever you want to tell me about yourself, and we can take all the time that we need to do that.

Analysis

The first and second responses that the therapist makes are similar; both are speaking to two sides of the split by acknowledging that they are both important parts of herself even though the patient wants to minimize one side of the split. The first responses points out that the patient's behavior is actually a form of communication, letting people know she's not fine. The second response allows for some distance from focusing on cutting as a bad thing. By inviting the patient to imagine what the cuts on her body might be trying to say both to herself and the people around her, she allows the patient to give voice so an action on a body level. The third response is more direct, using the authority of the adult in the room to make a declaration that the cutting behavior isn't "just fine." She lets the patient know that she values her enough to be concerned about her well-being. By declaring that she's not being judgmental, the firm, direct message coupled with a kind invitation allows the patient to feel the therapist's strength. It also gives tacit permission that the therapist's office she doesn't have to protect the adult in the room as she may have to do at home in an attempt to maintain some degree of family harmony.

Client Example Five

This client example involves the examination of splitting as a defense against grief and shame. The statement comes from a 70-year-old mother who had been bailing her son out of debt for years. This behavior has continued to enable his chronic pattern of drug abuse and under-employment. The therapist and client have been meeting off and on for several years whenever the mother reached a crisis with her son. The therapist's strategy in the past had been to offer suggestions, self-help books, and recommend that the patient attend Alanon. During a consultation group meeting, we discussed ways she might begin to speak to the split, exploring possible feelings of guilt and/or grief that were connected to the patient's ambivalence about setting firm limits with her son.

Patient Statement: **I guess I need to stop giving in to Johnny. I've been living with this for 10 years, and I've used up too much of my retirement money bailing him out. I know I need to do things differently. I just need to say no and stick with it. I was talking with my other son about all this, and he reminded me that Johnny knows that if he just keeps after Mom, she'll finally give in (pt. laughs). I know he's right; I just don't know why I keep doing it. (Face shifts to reveal sadness). I know the right thing to do, but I just want his asking to stop!**

Therapist Response Example #1: You said that you know the right thing to do, so I'm wondering what it is that interferes with your ability to say no to your son?

Therapist Response Example #2: What if he never stops asking? What do you think that would mean about him, and what would that mean about your relationship?

Therapist Response Example #3: I wonder, does your wish that he would stop asking you for money somehow get in the way of doing what you know you need to do? Are you hoping that he will somehow change, so you wouldn't have to act in a way that might disappoint him? Are you afraid that setting a limit with him will be the equivalent of abandoning him?

Analysis

The first response by the therapist looks to the side of the split that interferes with her ability to set a limit. This side of the split appears to be under-examined, even though she knows she's been unsuccessful. The patient feels a press from others to do the "right thing," but she seems to be less clear about the thoughts and assumptions that may keep her from taking action. The second response challenges the other side of the split by directly asking her to consider the possibility that he will never stop asking. Asking this simple, direct question can open a door to feelings of guilt over abandoning her son. In addition, by switching to the other side of the split, the therapist is inviting conversation about the patient's wishes and longings for her son to be different than he is. Her current behavior maintains her passive position in the relationship, loyally waiting for him to change without having to exert effort on her part. The third response speaks to both sides of the split by providing additional language to help frame and clarity to the patient's struggle. This may be useful in terms of helping the patient make connections. However, one of the risks in providing more language is that the therapist may be guided by her own assumptions rather than allowing the patient to reveal the material that has yet to come to the surface.

Client Example Six

The last example centers on a patient who entered therapy due to repeated indecisiveness in her workplace. Her pattern was to over-commit by vo-lunteering for assignments beyond her job description, which then created a situation where the patient became overwhelmed, unable to prioritize, and turn work assignments in on time. Whenever questioned by her boss or fellow teammates, she would become extremely ashamed and self-critical. Prior to the patient's statement below, the therapist had just reminded her that in the past she has been able to pick herself up, regather her strength and move forward.

Patient Statement: **I guess I do pick myself up after these dis-appointments happen, but it doesn't matter because it still hurts. If I were really strong, criticism wouldn't bother me. My mother taught us to be totally self-sufficient, to the point that I thought I should be able to figure out everything myself and not get frustrated or angry. Vulnerability doesn't really fit with that.**

Therapist Response Example #1: I'm wondering if your mother's expectations to be able to figure everything out by yourself is somehow connected to you not asking for help at work when you're feeling over-loaded. Did you ever consider that people at work might be willing to give a helping hand without seeing you as incompetent?

Therapist Response Example # 2: Why do you think being self-sufficient was so important to your mother? Did she teach you that strong, competent people never should feel vulnerable or have to ask for help?

Therapist Response Example # 3: You make it sound as if being vulnerable is a bad thing. Is it ever ok to feel soft and reach out for help? You're coming to me for therapy, and I'm wondering if that puts part of you in an uncomfortable position?

Analysis

The first response is aimed at breaking through the patient's assumption that challenge whether asking for help is a sign of incompetence. The therapist is speaking to the either/or split between strength being measured by not having needs vs. being needy as a sign of vulnerability and weakness. The second response asks a question that invites exploration of the family loyalty contract by examining mother's expectations more carefully. By asking the patient why self-sufficiency was so important, she allows the patient to question something that was never allowed to be questioned by her mother. The third response connects the patient's thoughts about exposing vulnerability as a bad thing to asking if there is a part of herself that feels uncomfortable asking for help from the therapist. This directs the conversation to examine the transferential feelings that may possibly be lying under the surface although not verbally expressed. Inviting this type of question is a form of permission-giving to process the enactment more consciously and verbally between them.

Statements that contain split-off material within any given therapy session eventually become enacted within the context of the therapeutic relationship. Entering into conversations about possible transferential enactments is a way to use the therapeutic relationship in the service of repairing dissociative splits. This topic will be covered in further detail in the next chapter.

Working with Unformulated Experience in the Clinical Hour

Many of the trainees in our consultation groups have difficulty knowing what stance to take with clients who have difficulty articulating a coherent sense of self in terms of goals, ambitions, feeling states and their desires in relation to others. When these clients are asked questions, there repeatedly seems to be a vagueness or paucity of language. There is also little differentiation between feeling states, as if the person in front of them appears lost or unformed. Our trainees describe the experience as hitting a wall or moving into empty space, where there seems to be very few verbal reference points for communication. Often client responses contain one-word answers, or they struggle with an inability to express an opinion or a feeling. It's as if there is no capacity for self-reflection, no way to even begin to articulate vague, amorphous feelings. When therapists try to engage these clients verbally, there is not only a paucity of words, but also a sense that the client is alone, embarrassed, lost, or confused.

At these moments in the dialogic process our trainees state that they, too, are at a loss and don't know what to say or do next. They feel pressured to do something, and many will try to over-compensate by asking more questions, offering suggestions, or making interpretations. One trainee described the experience as, "*I feel as if I've just entered La La Land.*" The phrase has stuck, and we use this to describe what it feels like for the therapist to be with clients where much of the personality seems to be unformulated or unknown.

Robert Grossmark (2018) describes patients who have difficulty formulating thoughts into verbal communication with another as being constrained, sometimes so severely, that they barely experience continuity of the self or any sense of subjectivity between self and others. He states,

"They may comply and utilize their verbal, related selves, but their inner core will remain at best untouched and at worst shamed into disavowal and inner sequestration" (p. 3) Individuals with either overly enmeshed and engulfing parental figures, or individuals who experienced severe deprivation, or individuals with dysregulated, inconsistent, or chaotic parental figures have difficulty clearly differentiating self from other.

When sensing the threat of separation or relational rupture another person's wishes or feeling states can create a blurring of identities. *"Is this my feeling or yours? When I try to speak up, everything gets numb and fuzzy, and I feel like I'm about to fall into a dark hole. It's just easier to go with the flow."* Or these individuals have difficulty expressing or identifying nuances of feeling states. They might respond, *"How do I feel? I don't feel much of anything. When I start to feel anxious, I just spend time in front of the TV or I play video games, sometimes for hours. When I wake up in the morning, I have this paralyzing feeling of dread. I don't know where it comes from."*

Donnel Stern states, "The unformulated is not yet knowable in the separate and definable terms of language. Unformulated material is composed of vague tendencies; if allow to develop to the point at which they can be shaped and articulated, these become the more lucid kind of reflective experience we associate with mutually comprehended verbal articulation." (Stern, 1997, pp. 37–38.)

Part of self-identity and mutual comprehension lies in the capacity to distinguish between self and other. Harry Stack Sullivan refers to the personified self as *me and not me*. He states that there is the good me and the bad me, and both parts of the self are what comprise the consciously recognized self. The *good me* is associated with positive feelings about self in the world, with praise and approval that is recognized consciously. The *bad me* includes aspects of the personality that an individual may not like, but they are more or less recognized consciously. The *bad me* is comprised of a person's worst, undesirable qualities, the parts of the self that engender feelings of shame that were internalized due to the fact that these parts of the self were met with disapproval from significant others. The *not me* represents parts of experience that exist within the self, but they never get symbolized.

Only in dissociation does *not me* exist. *Not me* is unformulated experience and exists completely outside of the client's awareness. Whereas the *bad me* is a conscious self-experience that individuals tend to avoid or hide because of intense feelings of shame and anxiety, the *not me* was treated as so unacceptable by the parent that it had to be split off from symbolic awareness. However, it remains alive in a segregated self-state, stored in the implicit memory system. The only way *not me* can be recognized within the treatment experience, and therefore brought forward, is by way of enactments. Donnel Stern (2010) equates *not me* states with a child's inability to "mentalize" experiences. Mentalization is the act of turning raw experience into symbolic form, and only when experience can be symbolized can it be carried in conscious awareness. Daniel Stern (1985) explains,

"Unformulated material is experience which has never been articulated clearly enough to allow application of the traditional defensive operations. One can forget or distort only those experiences which are formed with a certain degree of clarity in the first place. The unformulated has not yet reached the level of differentiation at which terms like memory and distortion are meaningful (p. 73)."

Donnel Stern (1997, 2009) summarizes by stating that unless or until the interpersonal field (through the therapeutic relationship) allows enough safety to formulate unsymbolized experiences, the not-me parts of the self will remain unformulated indefinitely. Of course, there are degrees or pockets of unformulated experience, depending upon the severity of the attachment injury. Proper assessment of the severity of attachment injury will determine the pace of the therapy dependent upon the client's capacity to move into a space of mutually comprehended verbal articulation. The greater the injury, the slower the unformulated parts of the self can be met with recognition and conscious awareness through acts of verbal articulation.

Client Illustration One

The following clip from a process recording illustrates a patient with an underdeveloped sense of self-awareness and/or the capacity to use language to express his inner world. The exchange that occurs between the therapist and the client reveals a greater and greater degree of shutting down as the therapist feels more lost in the unformulated space as he tries to offer questions or interpretations to fill what feels like the empty space between them.

Pt: *I guess right now I'm thinking about, um, like what grabbed my attention I guess that, like, I was feeling sort of like anxious I guess, about, or like uneasy about, I don't know, about talking about something. I mean something, something other than what were just talking about (laughs). Like, I don't know, I feel like the way we were just talking about that was like, I don't know. I don't know how to describe it, I guess.*

Th: *Well, that's okay. I mean, keep trying*

Pt: *(laughs, stares at the floor) 20 second pause.*

Th: *So, your mind just associated to feeling uneasy about things you and I were talking about?*

Pt: *Uh, no, no. It was like a break from what we were talking about. It's like I was just reflecting on this whole session, I guess. About how I feel, and how I didn't know how to bring something else up. Or if I wanted to bring something else up, and then I don't know.*

Th: *You mean like a new subject to talk about, or a new conversation topic?*

Pt: *Yeah.*

Th: *Was there something more important to spend our time with?*

Pt: *Yeah (tone changing) yeah, yeah. Basically. (laughs) But I don't know.*

Th: *Hum. Were there other things on your mind you were already conscious of wanting to talk about today?*

Pt: *Uh no, not really. I've been pretty busy today, I guess. I haven't had much time to think about it. I don't know, there's like a certain mood or mind state I have to enter into which is sort of like it was feeling, that I needed to enter into that space*

Th: *Ah, maybe that space where we go a little more into something that is more sensitive or a little more vulnerable?*

Pt: *silence*

Th: *Hum, and I felt like – well I definitely want your feedback – We did have one of those sessions last Tues where some new stuff came up. Is that what you want to talk about?*

Pt: *yeah, I guess, I don't know (long silence).*

Th: *I'm really glad you're trying to share this with me right now. I think it is good to hone in on something that came up before. It's like we can take a step back and try to talk about it together.*

Pt: *What do you mean?*

Th: *Like where we were on Tuesday, we can revisit what happened for you when we were in that more vulnerable territory.*

Pt: *(sounds a little confused) yeah?*

Th: *Did you have any reflections from that last session, between now and then?*

Pt: *(long pause) Um, no – I didn't.*

Analysis

Clearly, the patient is struggling to find words. He either has something to say but is afraid to say it, or he feels at a loss to know exactly what he is feeling or what it is that he needs from the therapist. Past sessions with the patient reveal a similar form of communication, where the patient struggles to find words or drifts into a dissociative stare when asked to describe feelings or sequences of events that trigger feelings. Ferro (2002, 2009) and Lombardi (2002, 2007) refer to patients who appear to interact in deadened, autistic-like states as an organization of experience where their felt sense of self is located in bodily sensations or symptom formation. In therapy the reliance on verbal articulation must be used with care so as not to overwhelm the patient with stimulation that exceeds the patient's capacity to assimilate and organize the information.

As you can see, the client example above does indicate an internal organizing schema that becomes easily flooded by over-stimulation. Therefore, it is recommended that engagement on the part of the therapist would initially involve less questioning of the patient as the therapist attempts to gain some form of a foothold of connection. Instead, the moment-to-moment unfolding within the treatment hour could allow for more silence on the part of the therapist in order to help the patient find his own pace of entering into the verbal and non-verbal exchange, a pace that allows space for the patient's own reverie and associations to emerge. Reis (2011) refers to this form of silence as a connected silence, a "with-ness" that doesn't intrude on the patient by introducing more than the he or she can experience in any given moment. (Lombardi, 2007) also suggests that it is initially helpful in working with these patients for the therapist to share his/her own "reverie," offering reflections of the felt sense of the dyadic experience. This can become a pathway into the emerging verbal narrative. However, Ferro (2009) cautions that with the use of language, there must be no active interpretative activity centered on the patient's internal world or on the relationship (p.14).

In this case scenario as the therapist began to back away from asking multiple questions one after the other, both parties began to become more comfortable with the slower rhythm of their interaction. Over time, the patient began to exhibit a bit more engagement in the therapeutic process. It wasn't that the patient was able to volunteer verbal information in a more articulated way, but the therapist described the atmosphere in the room as feeling less resistant on the part of the patient.

Later Session:

Th: *What would you like to focus on today?*

Pt: *I don't know, I didn't really have anything on my mind or a specific thing to talk about, I guess. I felt like, like noticed some like, uhh I don't know like avoiding trying to feel emotions this week.*

Th: *Mmm hmm.*

Pt: *Umm, like when I was a few days ago, I was like talking to Mary. I was like, really sad. She was like trying to get me to tell her what I was sad about and I was like, telling her that I was, like, hard to deal with. (Pause) Like breaking up with her and I was just like I don't know; I really don't want to talk about it. (Long Pause) I could just feel myself like, you know, not being able to even really think about it.*

Th: *Can you say more what that was like not being able to think about it?*

Pt: *Umm, it was like I was feeling really like really like strong emotions, like really sad and. It was like I couldn't like really put it into words, but I was upset.*

Th: *Mmm hmm.*

Pt: *It's like I couldn't really. And then I felt like I tried to think about it was kind of like a part of me was just like not going to like be willing to think about it like I don't know. So, a part of me was like trying to figure out what was going on, the other part was like running away from that thing.*

Th: *Can you say more about the running away feeling like? Was that a physical kind of thing?*

Pt: *No, it more just like thoughts, like there was one thought running behind another one.*

> (Pause). *Like one was trying to run away from the question. It was like trying to run away from that awareness. Sort of.*

Th: *Yes, so it sounds like you're feeling some pretty intense emotions and they were bubbling to the surface and as soon as they got there, part of you tried to maybe...* (Pt. interrupts)

Pt: *Yeah, I mean, it was kind of like I was like having like fleeting thoughts about, like what I was sad about. And then when I tried to like, really, like when Mary asked me about them, I tried to like, really like hone in on like one thing and I was not able to.*

Th: *Were there any of those thoughts that you want to open up with me, or would it be the same experience?*

Pt: *I don't know.*

Th: *Mm hmm. Yeah, does it feel like there's anything that you're aware of, but trying to hide so much is that it's just that things get very scrambled when you get to that point?*

Pt: *Yeah.*

Th: *I don't know if that...* (Pt. interrupts)

Pt: *Sort of, yeah.*

Th: *What would you add to that or what would you tweak?*

Pt: *Umm, I mean, that sounds right, I guess. I don't know, it was just so hard to describe, so. Just like not able to focus, really.*

Th: *Does it feel like when you try to describe those deeper, more vulnerable thoughts, that your emotion starts to become more intense?*

Pt: *Yeah.*

Th: *And you were aware of sadness, were you aware of anything else? Or were those her words?*

Pt: *No, those were mine.*

Th: *Mmm hmm.*

Pt: *Umm, mostly just sadness.*

Th: *Are you still feeling that way or is that feeling kind of and coming and going?*

Pt: *Like at the moment? No, not really.*

Analysis and Commentary

This session excerpt took place approximately nine months after the first transcript. You can see how the patient has made progress in both his verbal articulation and his attempts to reflect upon and track his own thoughts and feelings. There are even two occasions where he interrupts the therapist to further clarify what he is trying to say. The patient is able to describe that there was a part of him that *"was trying to figure out what was going on, and the other part was running away from that thing."* Even though he couldn't quite articulate what he was trying to run away from, he is able to express his newly forming reflective capacity. The therapist's next comment was to say, *"Can you say more about the running away feeling? Was that a physical kind of thing?"*. Here the therapist asks for clarification about one part of the patient's description and then moves to ask if it was a physical sensation.

This is an understandable next comment – to try to gather more information about the patient's avoidance. However, when we see movement toward integration of conflicting aspects of the self, a better response might have been to notice the growth within the patient's struggle and confusion. For example, a validating reflective comment might have been, *"I'm aware that you are now able to notice different parts of yourself. Are you aware of that? One part is trying to figure out the source of your sadness and there is another part of you that is afraid to go any further. This is important; it's real progress because before you would have just tried to push the feelings away."* This type of statement uses the therapist's words to create more of a container for understanding the internal world of the patient. These words convey both the therapist's awareness of the patient's interior self-states as well as giving the patient the sense that the therapist has joined him in those spaces.

Here is where a "serve and return" verbal response can further consolidate the patient's gains. This is what Donnell Stern (2019) refers to as the non-verbal "serving as a background for verbal meaning and thereby helping to establish the possibilities that exist for words, (p. 42)." This is also how observation followed by a reflective statement can capture the patient's struggle which in turn can play a role in the mentalization process. In this instance, the therapist verbally taking notice of the different parts of the patient that are beginning to emerge helps to reinforce the patient's observing self.

Later in the exchange the patient states that when he was trying to describe his thought process, he stated that one thought was running behind the other. A part of him was trying to run away from the question and another was trying to run away from self-awareness. This is one of the points in the session where the patient interrupts the therapist to finish what he was trying to say. *Pt: Yeah, I mean, it was kind of like I was like having like fleeting thoughts about, like what I was sad about. And then when I tried to like, really, like when Mary asked me about them, I tried to like, really like hone in on like one thing and I was not able to.* The patient is trying to communicate with the therapist that he was on the verge of being able to articulate *on his own* what he was sad about. He was trying to connect thoughts to feelings! When I read this process recording, I was reminded of watching an infant struggling with trying to take his first steps or in later childhood watching a child trying to figure out a puzzle. And when the parent tried to help, the child would push away the help and say, "No mommy, let me do it myself." And then, if the child later comes to the parent in frustration, the parent can then move to give assistance.

In this case when the patient gets to the place in the exchange where he goes back into his confusion (at the end of the transcription), the therapist can again offer verbal, reflective comments that summarize the process to help bring the non-verbal into verbal articulation. An example of such a statement might be, *"I know that this still feels like a struggle for you, but you're really describing this beautifully. We all have different parts of ourselves, and I heard you say that there are parts of you that want to be in touch with your feelings and parts of you that get confused or frightened. But that's sometimes just the way it is when we are learning about ourselves. It's so moving to be with you as you are becoming more aware of where you are in the process, and how well you are describing it. And I wonder what it feels like for you to hear me say that."* This reflective comment slows the process down and normalizes his discomfort. It is both reassuring and non-shaming. The therapist is also conveying in between the lines that just being able to name the dilemma brings the struggle into language in a way that can will help the patient begin to track his own thought processes.

When attempting to bring unformulated experience into conscious awareness, the goal for therapists is to try to slow our own mental processing down enough to be able to abide in the slower, quieter pace that is required to bring the unformulated into form. In this case when the therapist made this adjustment after the first transcript example, the patient was able to relax into the therapeutic holding environment without feeling pressured to respond verbally. As a result, less than a year later we see the patient's progress. He is beginning to demonstrate self-reflective capacities to the point that he is able to articulate his own internal conflict. In this transcript, you can *feel* how truthful he is being and how articulate he actually is becoming. When the therapist and supervisor processed this particular transcript together, the therapist said, "Ok, I get it. It's like he's struggling really hard to report data, and I'm putting it on a graph, so that we can both look at it." This is actually a simple and beautiful metaphor for capturing the complexity of the process dynamics required when bringing unformulated experience into verbal/symbolic representation.

Client Illustration Two

A second client example reveals a different pattern where pockets of unformulated experience appear to take over, flooding the patient to the point of momentary fragmentation. These types of patients may appear to be more well-constituted in terms of functioning in the world, to the point that they may even appear to demonstrate mutuality and inter-subjective connection. However, when triggered by fears of abandonment, prolonged states of emotional isolation, or when they feel pressured to express feelings of vulnerability, the therapist will often uncover pockets that the patients describe as places of emptiness, where the disconnected parts of themselves are experienced through a somatic or bodily sense that feels overwhelming. Balint (1968) refers to this state as the emergence of the most "primitive" parts of the patient's functioning, the places within the patient's fragility that become exposed within the treatment setting. If these hyper-aroused states are prolonged for any length of time, many patients will be triggered into a hypo-reactive, dissociative state of de-realization or depersonalization.

In this next case, we encounter a woman named Martha, who had been in individual therapy off and on for several years. Martha initially entered treatment prior to the birth of her first son due to feelings of anxiety at the thought of being an adequate parent. Therapy involved the exploration of family of origin issues that included a cold and distant mother, coupled with a father who had rigidly held beliefs about health, illness, and an overall disgust for human frailty. The patient reported that she never felt safe growing up. She was told that it was her fault whenever she became physically ill or had struggles with concentration in school. Her strategy was to try to become invisible at home and to excel in school so as not to experience her father's distain. During the course of therapy as the patient began to work on separating from her family's constant pressure and verbal criticism, her depression lifted, she became less timid and more confident as a mother, at which point she ended treatment.

Fifteen years later she reentered therapy due to struggles with her husband. The marriage had been a challenge in their earlier stages, but the birth of her son had given them a common focus. Now that Martha's son had grown, her sense of purpose was faltering. Marital tensions had increased over the years, and she now suspected her husband of having a secret affair. Much of the content of individual therapy was centered on her ambivalence about the marriage, and it was suggested that she and her husband also begin couples' treatment in concert with their individual therapies. Not long into couples' therapy, Martha began to complain of increased depression and anxiety. At times she reported extreme episodes of panic and withdrawal, largely centered on feeling invisible and ganged up on in the couples' therapy. Martha would leave these sessions stating that it often took her days to recover, where she felt confused and more alone. She was able to describe her experience in this way. "*It feels like I've fallen into the bottom of a well. Sometimes, I don't know who I am, if I really exist. I'm alone; it's dark, and there are no words to even make a sound to cry for help.*"

During this phase of treatment, the patient's depression increased, and she lost interest in outside activities. When her individual therapist asked the patient to describe what unfolded during the couple's sessions that made her feel so overwhelmed, she stated, "*I can't keep up with them. Larry talks so fast, throwing one topic out after another. He says that I'm angry and critical. How am I supposed to be honest when every time I try to say something, he gets wounded? The therapist encourages me to speak up, but when I do, I'm criticized for keeping score and blaming him.*" When the patient described her feelings of confusion and hopelessness to her individual therapist, she began to sob hysterically, stating that she didn't know if she had the strength to keep going on.

In a consultation with the couples' therapist, the couples' therapist described Martha being very flat, making little eye contact, and showing no emotion in the sessions. What seemed to trigger Martha's reactivity was when she perceived that her husband was asking for more from her. She somehow heard this as criticism, as if she wasn't enough. This when she seemed to shut down and had difficulty expressing herself in words. She stared at the floor and just shook her head.

At this point the individual and couples' therapist began to have regular check-ins to help manage the pace and timing of therapeutic interventions. Both therapists agreed that Martha needed to be given more room to process her thoughts and feelings within the couple's sessions. In an effort to help with verbalizing her thoughts, Martha and her individual therapist would discuss what she wanted to say and then rehearse and practice ways she could express herself. During these role-play sessions, the individual therapist was able to gain a window into identifying where Martha's reflexive assumptions around her own inadequacy were triggered. Together, they worked through ways she could challenge her assumptions by asking for feedback within the couples' therapy. The individual and couples' therapists also conferred about whether Martha's perceptions as to what happened in any given couples' session was in alignment with what the couple's therapist had observed. In this way, the individual therapist could work with Martha to help increase her sense of safety and to gently correct inaccurate assumptions, thus expanding the patient's window of tolerance. Over time, given the back-and-forth dialogue between the two therapists, Martha began to relax and feel safe within the couples' treatment which enabled the combined treatments to be more productive.

Summary

By focusing on splitting and dissociative self-states, this chapter spoke to several key elements that address the treatment of individuals who experienced the long-term effects of trauma and/or deprivation when left in prolonged states of dysregulation without the opportunity for relational repair. Research confirms that chronic, prolonged relational misattunement contributes to the development of dissociative splits within the personality that impact individuals well into adulthood. Neurological evidence and infant research have now directed us to rethink and expand our theoretical approaches to treatment when working with patient populations whose sense of self-coherence and self-regulation have been severely compromised.

In relationally based psychodynamic treatment approaches, we have witnessed a reexamination of how language is used as a communication tool. There has been a shift from a reliance on left-brain interpretations that resonate with patients' explicit memory processes to finding ways to connect with patients right-brain-to-right brain. This shift in approach involves observing and listening to our clients' experience in a way that attends to the nuances of non-verbal communication, including body language, eye contact, observing increases in agitation or abrupt decrease in connection that may reflect emotional shut-down. It is in these moments that we are able to see how unformulated self-states or implicit memory systems are brought into the room through non-verbal resonance. These are the places within our clients where there are no words, where simply being with our clients in these self-states of isolation and confusion is a form of companionship that is, in and of itself, a healing experience.

Finding ways to articulate these experiences in language creates a bridge to integrating emotion schemas that have been dissociated. Wilma Bucci (2011) explains that the reconstruction of emotion schemas occurs through a referential process that is held within the treatment relationship, allowing for sub-symbolic processes to be connected to symbolic representation in narrative and interactions within the session (Bucci, 2011). In this way implicit relational knowing can gradually begin to take shape in symbolic form. Bromberg (2006) had a similar view and explains that working with unconscious, procedurally organized aspects of relatedness that are outside the reach of symbolic representations, eventually will become organized into symbolic meaning through the relational experience that is created within the patient/therapist experience. Benjamin (2018) refers to this as "the rhythmic Third" and describes the aspects of procedural interaction that make intersubjectivity possible develops from the earliest mother-infant non-verbal exchanges of gesture, eye contact, and rhythmic cuing that make affective attunement possible. This requires right-brain-to-right-brain attunement.

Speaking to the splits is a doorway into understanding how to heal and integrate dissociated parts of the personality that can be accessed through symbolic representations. Asking questions about the parts of the whole that the patient may minimize or parts that may not align with current beliefs, feelings, or desires is a way of inviting the patient to become more curious and self-reflective. Speaking to the splits is a form of "mentalization" (Stern, 2010, 2019) that connects the dots by showing the inter-relationship between feelings, events, and memories that patients have yet to be able to connect on their own.

Having a trusted person to validate feeling states, name unfairness and trauma, support vulnerability to enhance the capacity to trust are all ways that split off parts of the self can be linked and connected to an ever expanding whole. As Peter Levine (2015) states, "The linking and processing of raw emotion, nuanced feeling, fact, and communication with chosen others is essential in moving from trauma—with a future barely different from the past—to an open future built upon new experiences, information, and possibilities, p. 17).

References

Balint, M. (1968). *The basic fault.* Tavistock.

Benjamin, J. (2018). *Beyond doer and done to: Recognition theory, intersubjectivity and the third.* Routledge.

Boston Change Process Study Group (2010). The foundational level of psychodynamic meaning: Implicit process in relation to conflict, defense, and dynamic unconscious. *Change in psychotherapy: A unifying paradigm.* Norton.

Bromberg, P. M. (1998). *Standing in the spaces: Essays on clinical process, trauma and.*

Bromberg, P. M. (2006). *Awakening the dreamer: Clinical journeys.* Mahwah, NJ: Analytic Press.

Bromberg, P. M. (2010). The nearness of you: Navigating selfhood, otherness, and uncertainty. In J. Petrucell (Ed.), *Knowing, not-knowing and sort-of-knowing: psychoanalysis and the experience of uncertainty* (pp. 23–44). New York: Routledge.

Bucci, W. (2011). The role of embodied communication in therapeutic change: A multiple code perspective. In W. Tschacher & C. Bergomi, (Eds.), *The Role of embodied communication in therapeutic change* (pp. 209–228). Imprint Academic.

Chu, J. (1998). *Rebuilding shattered lives: The responsible treatment of complex posttraumatic stress and dissociative disorders.* Guilford Press.

Crastnopol, M. (2015). *Micro-trauma. A psychoanalytic understanding of cumulative psychic injury.* Routledge.

Csikszentmihalyi, M. (2008). *Flow: The psychology of optimal experience.* Harper Perennial.

Danielian, J., & Gianotti, P. (2012). *Listening with purpose: Entry points into shame and narcissistic vulnerability.* Routledge.

DeYoung, P. (2015). *Understanding and treating chronic shame: A relational/neurobiological approach.* Routledge: Taylor & Francis Group.

Fisher, J. (2021). *Transforming the living legacy of trauma: A workbook for survivors and therapists.* PESI Publishing & Media.

Fischer, K. W., & Ayoub, C. (1994). Affective splitting and dissociation in normal and maltreated children: Developmental pathways for self in relationships. In D. Cicchetti & S. L. Toth (Eds.), *Disorders and dysfunctions of the self* (pp. 149–222). University of Rochester Press.

Ferro, A. (2002). *In the analyst's consulting room.* Routledge.

Ferro. A. (2009). *Mind works: Technique and creativity in psychoanalysis.* Routledge.

Goldberg, A. (1999). *Being of two minds: The vertical split in psychoanalysis and psychotherapy.* The Analytic Press.

Grossmark, R. (2018). *The unobtrusive relational analyst: Explorations in psychoanalytic companioning.* Routledge.

Horney, K. (1950). *Neurosis and human growth: The struggle toward self-realization.* Norton.

Howell, E. F. (2005). *The dissociative mind.* Routledge/Taylor & Francis Group.

Kernberg, O. (1975). *Borderline conditions and pathological narcissism,* Aronson.

Kestenberg, J. (1985). The flow of empathy and trust between mother and child. In E. J. Anthony & G. H. Pollack (Eds.), *Parental influences in health and disease* (pp. 137–163). Little Brown.

Kuchuck, S. (2021). *The relational revolution: In psychoanalysis and psychotherapy.* Confer Books.

Levine, P. A. (2015). *Trauma and memory: Brain and body in a search for the living past: A practical guide for understanding and working with traumatic memory.* North Atlantic Books.

Lyons-Ruth, K., Dutra, L., Schuder, M., & Banchi, L. (2006). From infant attachment disorganization to adult dissociation: Relational adaptations for traumatic experiences. *Psychiatric Clinics of North America, 29*(1), 63–86.

Lombardi, R. (2002). Primitive mental states and the body. *International Journal of Psychoanalysis, 83*, 363–381.

Lombardi, R. (2007). Shame in relation to the body, sex, and death: A clinical exploration of the psychotic levels of shame. *Psychoanalytic Dialogues, 17*(3), 385–399.

Putnam, F. W. (1989). *Diagnosis and treatment of multiple personality disorder.* Guilford Publications.

Putnam, F. W. (1997). *Dissociation in children and adolescents: A developmental perspective.* Guilford Press.

Reis, B. (2011, May). Silence and quiet: A phenomenology of wordlessness. [Panel presentation]. Annual Spring Meeting.: American Psychological Association, Division 39. New York.

Schore, A. N. (2012). *The science of the art of psychotherapy.* W. W Norton & Company.

Stern, D. (1985). *The interpersonal world of the infant.* Basic Books.

Stern, D. B. (1997). *Unformulated experience: From dissociation to imagination in psychoanalysis.* The Analytic Press.

Stern, D. B. (2009). Partners in thought: A clinical process theory of narrative. *Psychoanalytic Quarterly, 78*, 701–731.

Stern, D. B. (2010). *Partners in thought: Working with unformulated experience, dissociation, and enactment.* Routledge.

Stern, D. B. (2019). *The infinity of the unsaid: Unformulated experience, language, and the nonverbal.* New York: Routledge.

7 Working with Transferential Enactments as a Leverage for Change

Introduction

All unfinished business from the past is replicated in present-day relationships; all insecure childhood attachments inhibit the capacity for openness, curiosity, and full functioning. Using these two statements as anchoring points, the discussion of transferential enactments becomes the focus of this chapter. Unconscious, unarticulated, or disavowed material invariably becomes enacted in relationship to others, regardless of whether one *believes* in transference or has *proficiency* in using transference as a leverage for change. Transferential and counter-transferential dynamics occur in every therapeutic encounter. Clinicians who have not been trained to recognize potential transferential cues are at a disadvantage in terms of anticipating, managing, or working through these relational misattunements in the service of healing and repair.

"Transference *interpersonalizes* the patient's unconscious organizing schemas, schemas which lie at the heart of the patient's characterological structure. As such, transference constitutes an important cutting edge of therapeutic action, *a live here-and-now enactment* of important material not yet in awareness but edging closer to it. Therefore, as we create foundation stones of understanding, working with transference means working in the subjective present because, first and foremost, this is where the therapeutic dialogue becomes personal" (Danielian & Gianotti, 2012, p. 223).

Working with transference is one of the most powerful leverages for change at a therapist's disposal. As Robert Stolorow (2013) so eloquently states, "I have long contended that a good (i.e., a mutative) interpretation is a relational process, a central constituent of which is the patient's experience of having his or her feelings understood. Further, it is the specific transference meaning of the experience of being understood that supplies its mutative power, as the patient weaves that experience into the tapestry of developmental longings mobilized by the analytic engagement" (p. 377). In other words, it is through the unfolding therapeutic relationship that transference becomes the arena where unrequited longings are grieved,

DOI: 10.4324/9781003120278-8

prohibited anger and disappointment are expressed, and assumptions around trust and mistrust are worked through.

This chapter will provide examples as to how therapists can invite transferential exploration as well as how to anticipate and palpate the transference in hopes of mitigating and managing the complexity of potentially destructive negative transferential enactments. Transferential and counter-transferential reactions will be explored from the theoretical position of co-regulation and the intersubjective co-creation of "The Rhythmic Third" (Benjamin, 2018). Benjamin states that part of what makes intersubjectivity possible is a rhythmicity that is created through the early mother-infant relationship where a state of "oneness" is repeated with enough consistency that a state of affective attunement is established. It is this type of affective attunement created between the therapist and client that can lead to the repair of early attachment injuries.

In terms of contemporary psychodynamic views on transference, Benjamin is seen as providing a theoretical bridge between the classical approach to transference and the more contemporary relational schools. This bridge marks a shift, where the process of therapeutic engagement is seen as a co-creation of two subjective experiences that play out on the relational field. Laying the early groundwork for this shift was Sandor Ferenczi (1919, 1927), the first within the analytic community calling for a vital, honest responsiveness from the analyst toward the patient. His invitation has continued through the years with ever greater degrees of sophistication with the British Middle Group (Balint, 1968; Greenson, 1968; Winnicott, 1951, 1965; and Zetzel, 1970), and with more recent theoretical and neurobiological contributors who have directed their focus on the long-term impact of trauma and neglect. This expansion of our knowledge base has led to revisions in all of the analytic schools in terms of how one works with transferential and counter-transferential dynamics.

Among contemporary therapists, Robert Grossmark (2018) reminds us, "The treatment belongs to the patient, and it is the analyst's work to find and join with the register and wavelength that is the truest expression of the patient's inner world and experience. From this perspective, enactments are regarded as transpersonal narrations of what is beyond language and symbolization" (p. 3). He invites us to think about transferential enactments as the patient telling a story, one that can be conceptualized as narrations and representations in action that have yet to assume conscious, articulated form. Christopher Bollas (2009) points to the idea that human beings have a drive to *represent*, and the recognition of one's sense of self comes into being by being acknowledged by another. That which has not been recognized must be enacted before it can it assimilated into one's expanded sense of self. Robert Stolorow (2013) speaks of the intersubjective transferential interaction between the patient and therapist as that which allows for the expansion of the patient's reflective capacities, which in turn allows "the tight grip of old organizing principles to become loosened" thus increasing what can become 'nameable' within a context of human understanding and thereby enhancing and expanding one's very sense of being (p. 387).

The Importance of Working with Transference

Working with transference requires a belief that repeated relational patterns will eventually be projected onto the therapeutic stage, at which point the therapist will be pulled into the role of significant other and asked to engage in a complicated dance of idealization and de-idealization, a recreation of the patient's internal struggle between longing and mistrust. Therapists generally pick up on transferential cues through their own conscious and/or unconscious reactions to the patient over time. For example, feelings of being pressured, irritated, bored, or finding yourself having the need to be overly helpful are signs that transferential and counter-transferential material is being activated.

Working with transference also requires a belief that maintaining a benign, non-judgmental presence, in and of itself, can be powerfully healing and reparative. When the therapist creates a safe holding environment, the patient can experience being in relationship with another in a way that is mutual, respectful, and kind. In this way when a client brings transferential material into the room, the therapist has an opportunity to create an open, non-retaliatory relational response, a "lived" experience in the present moment. Taking the time to slow the process down, pausing to reflect upon and discuss process dynamics as they unfold, is what creates an opening for both client and therapist to explore unacknowledged feelings that have remained under the surface.

A patient's inability to articulate feelings verbally doesn't mean that he or she hasn't been activated transferentially. Bromberg (1998) explains that before "not-me" states of mind can become consciously recognized and reflected upon by the therapist and patient, they must first be communicated via enactments. When the therapist is able to verbally acknowledge the presence of transferential wishes, longings, and fears, a state of co-regulation and connection often follows. One way to look at transferential engagements is to consider them as representing the patient's greatest a state of "aliveness." It is through these enactments that the client is showing the therapist that which cannot yet be expressed in words. The therapist essentially serves as a witness and receiving station. Once this non-verbally enacted information is absorbed, it is the therapist's task to hold, metabolize, then translate into words that which could never be registered or expressed by the patient consciously.

Karen Maroda (2020) believes that transferential enactments are often a patient's best effort to communicate an important truth that was somehow forbidden to be acknowledged consciously. Most of what could never be registered consciously by the patient becomes sequestered in self-states that were either forbidden to be expressed or treated with disgust on the part of the parent. Therefore, these relational experiences remain stored in self states that are disavowed, filled with feelings of shame, waiting to erupt in the form of negatively charged transferential enactments. When optimally used, negative transferential experiences of rupture and repair can result in a sense of understanding and relief on the part of patients, where they feel seen and understood, rather than judged or shamed.

Because transference is the portal that connects prior wounds to present-day enactments, this window of understanding enables the therapist to see how early attachment injuries (the rules contained in learned loyalty contracts) manifest in relationship. Transferential enactments *always* telegraph information to the therapist. What is split off or dissociated eventually becomes enacted in the transference. Therapists register these split-off parts of the patient's psyche both consciously, in the form of their clinical observations and reflections, as well as unconsciously, through their corresponding counter-transferential feelings and responses.

There is no better way to understand the quality of a patient's early attachment patterns and learned loyalty contracts than by being on the receiving end of a relational enactment. In my view transferential enactments have a way of penetrating time and space because it is when we are able to resonate with the felt sense of being with our patients that we are better able to imagine what inner struggles and fears they carry. When patients *tell us about* their suffering and frustrations, this is one step removed relationally speaking because the patient is telling us about the experience, not engaging in the experience with us. In instances where transferential enactments become activated, therapists have an opportunity to approximate more closely what it feels like to be in the patient's skin.

The aim of any transferential dialogic exchange is to open a doorway to engage the client's curiosity as to new possibilities for connection. This is done by providing reassurance, correcting misunderstandings, or giving permission for negative reactions to be present without the patient having to experience retaliation on the part of the therapist. It is only when the therapist treats the patient differently than s/he expects that the patient can then experience a new way of being in relationship with another. This, in turn, gives patients an opportunity to challenge their own automatic assumptions, thus mitigating reflexive fears of disappointment. As a result, patients have an opportunity to disengage from patterns that had prevented them from accessing support from others in the past. It is through the processing of enactments and reenactments that a more benign experience of being in relationship is slowly able to become internalized as past relational failures gradually become ameliorated by successful, present-day relational exchanges.

Part of the success in working with transferential enactments as a means of creating relational repair is dependent upon the therapist's ability to remain steady. This is primarily done by adopting a stance that is non-judgmental and non-retaliatory, continually giving permission for the patient's real self to emerge. Therapeutic engagement is an intersubjective interaction which is also based on the acceptance that our presence can never be perfectly neutral or benign. Because we are fallible human beings with our own relational (counter-transferential) blind spots and biases, it is this aspect of working with transference that makes entering into the transferential arena a bit unsettling.

From a sociocultural standpoint, Brown, 2017, 2019; Brickman, 2018; Leary, 2000; and Myers, 2011; draw our attention to cultural attitudes and unconscious assumptions toward race and racial difference that have created clinical blind spots that have the potential to create "racial enactments" between client and therapist. Long et al. (2020) studied racial differences in the process of rupture and repair between Black patients and their White psychoanalytic therapists and found that therapists often failed to identify moments of rupture, particularly in the area of racial difference. From the patient's perspective, they powerfully described feelings of avoidance, silence, shame, hate, and racial identifications and disidentifications.

Jessica Benjamin (2018) points out the importance of therapists being able to acknowledge their role when failures of attunement occur or when their own unconscious triggers contribute to patient's resulting injuries. When patient and therapist are able to process what contributes to ruptures on any level, both parties can reestablish safety, which in turn can help repair the harm that may have been created by the co-participation in unconscious enactments or cultural blind spots.

Donnel Stern (2010, 2015) invites therapists to adopt a willingness to enter into an intersubjective space with our patients, where we allow ourselves to be open to our patients' "dissociated impact on us." He explains that this is how we are able to feel and experience the patient's unrepresented (unsymbolized) experience, and in turn reflect those memories and experiences back to them. In other words, working intersubjectively within the transference and counter-transferential exchange is how the conversion of pre-reflective, procedural experience can be turned into consciously experienced symbolic thought. Botella and Botella (2005) describe the act of entering into this type of intersubjectively experienced transferential space as allowing ourselves to become our patients' "doubles," as if we are able to experience the patient's mind from the inside. In doing so we are better able to verbally articulate the patient's unrepresented experience back to them in a way that helps establish meaning and allows the patient to be seen and understood.

The use of language, translating unconsciously enacted material into verbal meaning, is not the only way to hold and work through transferential episodes that become manifest during treatment. Robert Grossmark (2016) believes that true healing and therapeutic repair "often involves going further *into* our patients' worlds of suffering and private madness rather than working to move them *out* of these states" (p. 699). For patients where there is no capacity for mutuality or no differentiation of self and other, the use of language and symbolization to help soothe or repair are greatly limited, if not ineffective. It is in these situations that the therapist must act as a companion, entering into the dark "archaic" areas of functioning rather than seeking to foster greater relatedness in the session.

Margaret Black (2003) states that there is nothing more powerful than sitting through and surviving an intense explosion of affect during a session without feeling pressed to impose language. Simply holding the affect without retaliating or using words to explain the experience may convey non-verbally that the therapist is sturdy enough to weather emotional storms, demonstrating that the patient's emotions will not destroy either party nor the therapeutic connection.

As an illustration of this, a client of mine recently began his session by relating an event that occurred at his workplace. He began by speaking in an even tone, reporting the facts that transpired with a co-worker, explaining why he thought he had been treated disrespectfully. Suddenly, he jumped up from his chair, yelling and waving his finger in the air in frustration. His eyes had a look of rage, and spit was literally flying from his mouth when he spoke. When he finished, he sat down, breathing heavily, and glared at me. I simply returned his gaze without saying a word. Eventually, I began to slowly nod my head. The silence lasted for several moments at which point I noticed his whole body begin to relax. It was at this point that I asked him if he had anything more that he wanted to say. He smiled, and it was then that we were able to begin to process what had occurred. My sense was that the patient didn't experience a sense of shame, nor did he feel the need to apologize. It felt as if he knew he had revealed a forbidden part of himself that had been waiting to be released for years. As we sat in that silent space together, a sense of acceptance and conscious witnessing had occurred be-tween us. We had weathered the storm without either party being harmed. Here is how not rushing to find words is sometimes just as important as translating what is unknown into verbal meaning.

In sum, working with transferential enactments requires an emotional sturdiness on the part of the therapist that includes a willingness to engage in honest reflection. This involves using our own subjective experience as a barometer to, a.) reflect upon and eventually put into words the dy-namic that is being created between us, as well as b.) using our own self-awareness as a means of differentiating our own unconscious triggers from what we are receiving from our client's projected assumptions about us. In the broadest sense, relational psychotherapy has shifted its position regarding the successful working through of transferential dynamics, placing more emphasis on context and the co-creation of the therapeutic experience. No longer viewing the therapist as the objective, neutral expert, the relational position asks therapists to enter into an inter-subjective experience, where self-examination and clinical supervision are as important as learning a theory or mastering a technique.

Inviting Clients into Transferential Dialogue Through Listening for Entry-Point Cues

One way to listen for possible transferential cues is by paying attention to entry-points in the client's language. Trainees that are new to the process of working with transference often ask how they can know that a patient's statement holds a transferential meaning or if they're just making conversation. The answer is that we don't know for sure, but it doesn't hurt to explore the possibility. Often seemingly innocent or benign statements convey assumptions that will eventually be placed onto the therapist as a transferential enactment. Also, over-generalizations of any kind are likely to convey a transferential communication.

Here are some possible transferential statements that often fly under the radar of therapeutic inquiry. If we hear them as actual entry points, these statements represent the tip of the iceberg of communicating something more dimensionally complex. Often these types of statements telegraph a patient's underlying feelings of shame or inadequacy. They may also convey their longings for rescue or fears of being disappointed.

- "People are like the weather. You can never know what's coming next."
- "How can you really ever trust anybody? They all leave sooner or later."
- "I feel more comfortable with animals than I do people."
- "You're really smart. Most people can't keep up with me."
- "Of course, I'm fine. I've always been able to take care of myself."
- "Why do you keep asking me how I'm feeling? Feelings are overrated."
- "Can't you just tell me what to do to help fix this chaos?"
- "Your office is the only safe place."
- "I wish that I could just run away."
- "I hope you won't think I'm crazy for saying this…"
- "I don't know why you are charging me for that appointment I missed. I told you I was sorry. Don't you ever make a mistake?"

As you listen for the transferential meaning in these entry point phrases, notice repeated themes that may express frustration, over-determined efforts, fear of judgment, or longings for rescue. When you are able to identify a repeated theme, this provides a window into the patient's potential feelings about the therapy or the therapist, including internalized assumptions about the power differential that is created when any client seeks help from an "expert." When struggles around power, control, and vulnerability are expressed, feelings of shame and the fear of domination or exploitation are often under the surface. For example:

- At times the therapeutic power differential may be expressed through the theme of **control or fear of loss of control coupled with an indirect challenge**, as in the two example statements – "*Of course, I'm fine. I've always been able to take care of myself,*" and "*Why do you keep asking me how I'm feeling? Feelings are over-rated*"
- At other times the power differential may be conveyed in the form of **over-idealizing the therapist or wishing that someone will provide rescue from a problem**, as exemplified in the phrases – "*Can't you just tell me what to do to help fix this chaos,*" or "*Your office is the only safe place,*" or "*I wish I could just run away.*"
- Finally, statements that signal a struggle over power dynamics often manifest in the form of **fear of negative judgment or fear of being taken advantage of** as exemplified in the statements – "*I hope you won't think I'm crazy for saying this...*" or "*I don't know why you are charging me for that appointment I missed. I told you I was sorry. Don't you ever make a mistake?*"

In addition to listening for entry points that convey hidden feelings about the tension around power, domination, and shame, the themes of trust and mistrust are also a doorway into transferential exploration. The first three entry point comments listed above are all examples of statements that telegraph some degree of relational mistrust - "*People are like the weather. You can never know what's coming next,*" "*How can you really ever trust anybody. They all leave sooner or later,*" or "*I feel more comfortable with animals than I do people,*" are over-generalizations that convey relational meaning.

Generalized statements don't enter the therapeutic dialogue simply because the client is trying to make small talk. Whenever a patient makes a statement that conveys an assumption about relationships, it is prudent to wonder what might be happening between the therapist and the client in that moment. Is the client letting the therapist know that he can't let his guard down? Is he saying he can't rely on her to not eventually disappoint him, or that he's afraid she'll get frustrated with him and end treatment prematurely? When therapists ask for clarification about statements that convey an assumption about relationships, this is how an opening can be created that uncovers transferential feelings and/or assumptions. Furthermore, asking for clarification is a form of permission-giving, a way of letting the client know that it's ok to talk about the feelings that come up as the therapeutic process unfolds.

When in doubt as to whether a statement conveys transferential meaning, a general rule of thumb is – if there is a history of neglect and/or shame coupled with a pattern of over-determined self-sufficiency, the likelihood of a transferential enactment is high. For example, when the patient's entry point phrase makes a reference to women or men in a way that expresses a bias along gender lines or socio-economic status, this may have particularly significance transferentially. When patients express feelings of being stuck or bored with life, they may be indirectly communicating that the therapy is at an impasse. If clients express a devaluing of self or others, it is likely that they fear being negatively judged by the therapist.

As you move into inviting transferential engagement, ask yourself the following questions:

• How aware is the patient of repeating patterns in their relationships?
• How does the patient react to you when you point out repeated patterns?
• What is their degree of self-reflection, curiosity?
• What is their degree of minimization?
• What is their degree of defensiveness?

The patient's reaction to you when you point out patterns in other relationships will determine the likelihood of a transferential enactment occurring with you at some point in the treatment process.

Client Example

Chapter Four provided a client example where the tracking of the entry-point dialogue could have led to a possible transferential exploration. The initial therapist/client exchange is provided below. However, the therapist could have easily chosen to invite questions that may have revealed a transferential communication just under the surface. As you read this exchange again, notice the statements that are bolded. They are potential openings for inquiry about something that the patient may be experiencing about the therapist.

Pt: *"You and I both know that my wife tends to over-react."*
Th: *"What do you mean, over-react?"*
Pt: *"Well you know, I've talked about this before."*
Th: *"Could you give me an example of something that happened this week where she over-reacted?"*
Pt: *"She got upset because I forgot to take out the trash, but I had a really hectic week, and I was out of town and came in late. I don't know why she couldn't be more understanding."*
Th: *So, you were hoping she'd be more understanding? What did that feel like when she wasn't?"*
Pt: *"Like I said, I shouldn't be surprised. She always over-reacts.* **I guess all women are a little too emotional.**"
Th: *"So, you handled your disappointment with your wife by telling yourself that all women are a little too emotional? Don't you have a right to feel disappointed?*

Pt: *"I know I shouldn't lump all women into the same category. You're right, I was disappointed, and I was a little angry if you must know. Sometimes it makes me feel hopeless that she'll ever really be there for me."*

Th: **"And that feeling of hopelessness makes you tell yourself that all women are too emotional. Does that make you feel less angry with your wife?"**

Pt: *"Yes, it's what makes me keep hanging in there. I guess I tell myself, what's the point in making a fuss. **All women are just so sensitive. It's easier to keep my mouth shut.**"*

Th: *"How is that easier?"*

As you review the above dialogue, what thoughts went through your mind when you read the statement, "I guess all women are a little too emotional." "All women" is an over-generalization that may be a tip-off that the patient is having a similar emotional reaction to his female therapist. Even if the patient is not aware of it in the moment, it is likely that at some point in time the patient will eventually experience some form of fear that the therapist won't be able to tolerate his feelings or his needs. A second statement that conveys the same generalization is the patient's last statement, *"All women are just so sensitive. It's easier to keep my mouth shut."* In this statement the patient is giving further clues that he is likely to be hesitant to speak about any discomfort he may be experiencing in the therapy. This reenactment may take the form of over-protecting the therapist's feelings or withholding important information from the therapeutic exchange.

These statements give the therapist an opportunity to explore the patient's feelings and assumptions about women more thoroughly *before* an enactment actively surfaces between them. For example, the therapist may wish to inquire whether there were any times in the therapy where the patient decided not to speak up when he felt uncomfortable or disagreed with the therapist. *"Has there ever been a time between us where you thought it might be easier to just keep your mouth shut rather than speak up?"* Asking this question in response to the patient's statement about his wife is a way of anticipating an enactment that is likely to play out between the therapist and patient in the future. By anticipating and naming the possibility that a similar reaction may occur in the treatment, the patient is being given permission to verbalize those feelings without the fear of recrimination.

In terms of the timing as to when to invite a discussion about the patient's reactions to the therapist or the therapy depends on the patient's level of comfort with the process. In a general sense, when you sense that there might be a transferential/counter-transferential reaction that is taking place between you, it is better to gently open the dialogue up for exploration sooner rather than later. Palpating possible transferential cues early on in the treatment is a way of letting the patient know that it's ok to share less than positive feelings about the therapeutic experience. It is also a way to explore possible negative reactions before they build up into overall mistrust without the micro-attunements that lead to repair.

Understanding Transference as the Enactment of Two Sides of a Split

In Chapter Six we discussed how splitting can often represent a reenactment of posttraumatic dominant-submissive relational patterns, where the child internalizes the experience of being in relationship based on being on the receiving end of an abusive, often rageful and/or neglectful caregiver. The result is the organization of self in relation to other becomes split apart along the axis of relational trauma, into two alternating self-states – the helpless victim self-state and (the often less conscious) abusive/rageful self-state (Howell, 2005).

The development of healthy self-agency and the capacity for mutuality and interdependence requires mirroring and validation, the "serve and return" where the child is given the freedom to articulate wishes and desires as well as having the experience being able to influence important others. Children who grow up in traumatic, dominant-submissive relationships have no opportunity to share their feelings and desires, no ability to modify the aggressor's behavior to accommodate the child's plea to be seen and understood as an independent being. Because no experiential memory of separateness and interdependence could develop, the two self-states of victim and aggressor could not be integrated into a sense of the whole self. They had to remain rigidly split off from one another.

Often clinicians become confused by clients who present as victims, only to find that eventually they are on the receiving end of the patient's relentless demands coupled with accusations of not feeling properly understood or valued. Elizabeth Howell (2005) explains these types of enactments are a replication of the traumatic relationship that was experienced in childhood, where the child orients around the aggressor from the victim position, yet procedurally learns and unconsciously mimics or enacts the aggressor position as a result of the intense attachment that was formed. Therefore, in adult life an individual may identify as a kind and giving person who is often taken advantage of by others; however, the dissociated aggressor position is enacted in relation to others in response to not having his/her needs met. Jessica Benjamin (2019) explains that for therapists being on the receiving end of a dissociated, aggressive enactment, it often feels as if there is something that's coming at us that is "just too much." For example, when a patient accuses the therapist for making her feel guilty, it's not that the guilt is too difficult to hold, Benjamin states. The hardest part is holding the dissociative enactment without becoming flooded or confused.

In clinical situations unarticulated (unformulated) enactments are often experienced counter-transferentially as something coming at us that feels too much, too intense. The patient's feelings are dissociated, but they live relationally in a realm where there is no differentiation between self and other. Benjamin states that as therapists when we feel flooded, we may have lost our capacity for differentiation, and thus are unable to reestablish the Rhythmic Third, which is the ability to soothe and reestablish non-verbal attunement. When patients engage in a transferential enactment, the state of rhythmicity between patient and therapist is off, or as she states, the music and the lyrics are completely off. Benjamin advises that when there is a rupture, what is of primary importance is the need to return to the flow or the rhythmicity of connection. To unpack the enactment in all its gory details, doesn't always necessarily need to happen initially. However, eventually the "not me" part of the self that wishes to do harm (like the aggressor did harm to the child) needs to be brought to the surface and processed consciously.

Client Example

The next client example illustrates aspects of the "not me" parts of self that have become activated within the dialogue between therapist and client. This activation is marked by sudden, extreme shifts in the client's affect that bring the dissociated aggressor part of the self to the surface. In the three dialogic exchanges below, the client repeatedly becomes defensive whenever the therapist makes a reflection or asks a question. Each example reveals a slightly different defensive response, but all responses reveal the client's need to reestablish a sense of control by retaliating when he assumed that there was a negative judgment contained within the therapist's question.

As you read these case excerpts, you will notice that the therapist didn't stop the conversational flow to wonder what may have triggered the patient's aggressive emotional response. Instead, he tried to smooth the waters to avoid increasing the patient's irritation. The therapist disclosed that this had been an intentional choice. His objective was to return to the flow or the "rhythmicity" of the connection to strengthen the therapeutic alliance. However, in a later consultation session the therapist also admitted that he sometimes felt intimidated by the patient, a locally famous professional actor who was quite a bit older than the therapist.

Three brief dialogic interactions are provided below where each of the client's responses exemplify a similar pattern of reactivity. As you read through them, try to identify what transferential themes are beginning to emerge. Also, try to imagine what you might have said that would have impacted the direction of conversation moving forward. Following each example, an alternative response as well as an analysis will be provided as to what the therapist could have said to explore the underlying transferential enactment further.

Background: This 62-year-old patient grew up with a verbally abusive, critical father and an anxious, overly doting mother. The patient has been reluctant to discuss his past history at any point in the therapy. Instead, the majority of the patient's discourse revolve around complaints about his marriage. He states that he chronically feels victimized and taken advantage of by his wife but is at a loss because he doesn't want to hurt her. The patient sees himself as a giving and patient man, but he essentially feels that his wife is unappreciative and preoccupied with her own physical health or her civic non-profit commitments. The patient also has a work history marked by ruptured relationships, where he had been given feedback that he was "domineering and unreasonable." In one instance he was even involved in a lawsuit for sexual harassment. His response to this feedback was to become enraged and blame others for being too sensitive or narcissistic. During the course of treatment, the therapist reported that whenever he tried to direct the patient to focus on familial factors that may be connected to his ambivalence, or past disappointments in other relationships, the patient would either go on a rant about the lawsuit or become dismissive of family-of-origin factors that may have relevance in his present struggles with his wife.

Exchange Number One: For weeks the client had explained in detail how he would continue to bend over backwards trying to please his wife but would never receive any appreciation or praise. As a way of following up on the theme of lack of reciprocity, the therapist offered the reflective comment:

Th: "*You give so much of yourself to your wife, and you seem to get nothing in return.*"

Pt: (Agitated with raised voice) "*Hey, I don't need you to criticize my wife, I'll be the one to do that.*"

Th: (Taken aback) "*I didn't mean to criticize her. I was just trying to remind you that we've been talking about how you seem to vacillate back and forth between how you feel about her.*"

Pt: (Becoming calmer and smiles) "*Well, you'd better not do it again. I'm the only one who has a right to complain. You're not married to her.*"

Alternate Response: After this brief exchange, the therapist reported that he didn't make a comment about the patient's outburst stating that he was afraid to challenge him because he didn't know what to say without creating more tension between them. Rather than initially offering an apology by saying that he didn't mean to criticize her, an alternative way that the exchange might have unfolded could look like this:

Th: "*You give so much of yourself to your wife and you seem to get nothing in return.*"

Pt: (Agitated with raised voice) "*Hey, I don't need you to criticize my wife, I'll be the one to do that.*"

Th: "*I'm sorry. Did you hear me criticize your wife just now?*"

Pt: "*Yeah, you said she gives me nothing in return. Are you saying she's selfish?*"

Th: "*No, not at all. I was just repeating what you had said to me. Do you remember saying those words?*

Pt: "*Yes, of course I do, but that doesn't mean you get to say it.*"

Th: "*I'm wondering what is it about hearing someone else mention your own words that made you have such a reaction? I'm wondering how I could help you explore all of your feelings about your wife, all of your needs without you feeling that you have to protect her or defend her in front of me, especially when you express your own dissatisfaction?*"

Analysis

In this client example, the therapist begins the exchange by directly asking if the patient *heard* him criticize his wife. This puts the ball back into the patient's court in terms of inviting him to consider that he may have possibly misunderstood the therapist. This question then prompted the patient to assume that the therapist thought his wife was selfish. Once this assumption was exposed, it gave the therapist an opportunity to reassure the patient to correct the negative assumption. However, the patient wasn't appeased and re-asserted his need to establish control by challenging the therapist more directly, ordering him not to speak about his wife in negative terms. Clearly, the aggressor self-state is now at the surface, and it becomes easier to see how the patient is replaying a theme of dominance and subservience within the dyad. In an effort to break this pattern, the therapist gives the patient permission to have the control by asking the patient how he can better help him explore his feelings and needs.

This takes the therapist out of the role of either being the victor or the victim, hopefully reestablishing attunement.

Exchange Number Two: In this scenario the therapist begins the session by picking up on a statement the patient had made shortly before the end of the session the previous week. The patient had stated that he felt trapped in his marriage and was thinking of asking for a separation.

Th: "*I wanted to get back to something you had said at the end of our session last week. You mentioned that you were feeling trapped in your marriage.*"

Pt: (Interrupts) "*Hey buddy. Let me get this straight. I DO NOT feel trapped. I can leave any time I want to.*"

Th: "*Oh, I'm sorry, I must have misheard you. What were you trying to say last week?*"

Pt: "*That's ok. I was trying to say that I didn't want to attend her big social event. I knew I was going to be bored out of my mind. And as it turns out, I was.*"

Th: "*Well, what was it that made you bored?*"

Alternate Response: In this exchange the therapist has a couple of options as to when to comment on the patient's agitation around feeling accused of being trapped. He could pause and immediately comment on the intensity of his response, or he could wait to see how the patient reacted after his apology and his request for clarification. I actually think that the therapist's apology was a good next response because it might have diffused the affective charge while keeping the exploration open in order for the therapist to ask further clarifying questions. However, when the patient quickly moves away from the affective intensity of his response and switches to talking about being bored at his wife's social event, the next comment from the therapist needs to circle back to what just happened between them a moment ago. A possible intervention that the therapist could have made is as follows:

Th: *"Wait just a minute. Before we begin to explore your feelings about being bored at your wife's event, can we talk about what just happened between us?"*

Pt: *"What do you mean?"*

Th: *"You seemed to become angry when I mentioned the phrase 'feeling trapped'. It almost seemed as if you thought I was accusing you of being weak or being something that you're not."*

Analysis

This type of intervention directs the patient to look at the effect that his words may have on other people. It also named the possible affect under the surface while simultaneously asking whether the patient actually felt accused of being weak or inadequate. By naming this aloud, this helps the patient put language to an emotion as well as what might possibly have triggered the emotion. Holding this conversation in conscious awareness between them creates the opportunity process the relational interaction more openly.

Exchange Number Three: In this vignette, the client demonstrated what seemed to be two contradictory behaviors that stood out to the therapist. At the end of the session the prior week the patient announced that all he ever talked about in the therapy was his wife, and he wanted to shift the focus to himself moving forward. As the patient entered into this session, he again proceeded to spend the majority of his time complaining about his wife. The therapist, remembering the patient's request from the prior week wanted to shift the focus back to the patient. The therapist then engaged in the following exchange.

Pt: *"She constantly complaining about something being wrong with her physically but she won't go to the doctor. It's all psychosomatic."*

Th: *"Do you ever struggle with psychosomatic issues yourself?"*

Pt: (Looks up). *"I went to four different clothing stores before picking one."*
Th: *"Where did you end up going?"*
Pt: (Shaking his head), *"I'm not going to tell you."*
Th: *"Why not?"*
Pt: *"You wouldn't know anyway."*

Alternate Response: The therapist is trying to hold both sides of the split; however, he ends up following the sequence of the content of the conversation, rather than finding a way to articulate his dilemma with regard to the patient's conflicting messages. An alternative way to hold the dilemma could be the following.

Pt: *"She constantly complaining about something being wrong with her physically, but she won't go to the doctor. It's all psychosomatic."*
Th: *"I remember at the end of last session you told me that you wanted to spend more time focusing on yourself. So, I'm wondering how you want me to respond to your concern about your wife right now? Is this the most important thing you wish to bring forward today?"*

Analysis

This statement, made at the beginning of the session, is a way for the therapist to not only speak to the split, but it allows him to share his dilemma with the patient without being put in a double bind. By asking the patient how he would like the session to proceed gives the control back to the patient as well as reminding him of his responsibility to follow through on what he had requested last week. The patient may have not remembered what he said the previous week, but the therapist mentioning it brings continuity into the session. It also conveys that even if the patient cannot remember, the therapist is able to hold the entire picture in between sessions.

When therapists fail to hold the big picture and reflect the continuity of the dynamic from session to session, there is a greater likelihood that further enactments will occur. As we can see this is what happened when the patient began to talk about going to four clothing stores. When the patient made this puzzling shift in the dialogue, the therapist had another opportunity to remark on the process dynamic that was unfolding, rather than again staying with the content of asking the patient which store he picked. As a means of tracking the process, the therapist could have said something like this, *"I'm sorry, I'm a bit confused. I'm not sure how going to four clothing stores connects with your concerns about you or your wife being psychosomatic?"* Notice that when the therapist stayed with the content, the patient became either more withholding or more irritated when he said, *"I'm not going to tell you."* Here we see an openly direct challenge that is directed to the therapist. The enactment continues to be played out between them rather than being processed and understood.

Attunement, Misattunement, Repair

No matter how much patients desire our help, there is a part of them that enters therapy not believing that help is really possible. For patients with a history of trauma, Bessel van der Kolk (2015) explains that trauma results in a fundamental reorganization of the way mind and brain manage perceptions. Trauma is not just an event that took place in the past. It is also the imprint left by that experience on the mind, brain, and body (p. 21). In other words, trauma is an involuntary restructuring of the brain that creates an experience of permanence in their emotional reactivity. What kind of reactivity? What therapists are able to observe is a variation in the band width of a patient's "window of tolerance." From the client's perspective, trust and mistrust are hard-wired reactions based on early attachment failures. Additionally, from the client's perspective, this is considered "normal," and can be recognized by statements such as, *"This is just who I am, and I have always been this way." "It is just the way it is."* Trust and mistrust are not based on present moment experiences. Rather, they are learned reflexive responses based on early emotional imprinting due to chronic attachment failures.

These early imprints, stored in the brain's representational networks, will determine which attachment state will be most often activated and repeated, thus affecting the quality of one's relationships throughout life (Cozolino, 2002, 2006; Lyons-Ruth, 1999, 2003; Wallin, 2007). Janina Fisher (2021) describes clients who suffer from a wide range of attachment injuries that affect the wiring of the brain, as "the living legacy of trauma," and she states,

> One of the many consequences of trauma is a loss of trust in human beings. Fear of vulnerability, a phobia of dependence, fear of self-disclosure, and careful avoidance of sadness and anger are also common symptoms. Each of these fears is adaptive in a world in which even a child's caretakers are not to be trusted, where tears or anger are punished, emotional needs are exploited, and dependence is dangerous (p. 2).

As therapists, we understandably want our clients to trust us. But as van der Kolk (2015), Fisher (2021), Lanius et al. (2014) explain that patients with trauma histories are more easily dysregulated because their affective window of tolerance is much narrower. Therefore, they are frequently triggered to enter into states of hyper-arousal or hypo-arousal. As a result, the patient's ability to trust in others is highly compromised. Treatment must involve learning new patterns of regulation using both the mind and the body in the healing and recovery process where attention needs to be given to learning new patterns of regulation and co-regulation.

Initially, the therapist must act as a moderator or the executive functioning part of the patient's brain because the window of tolerance is so

narrow. Efrat Ginot (2009) explains, "An environment suffused by emotional stress and compromised soothing in early childhood will result in
frequent activation of the fear system and automatic defenses meant to
minimize the viscerally experienced stress" (p. 294). Allan Schore (2012)
states that the therapist must act as an auxiliary cortex and affect regulator of
the patient's dysregulated states.

By providing an atmosphere within the therapeutic relationship that is
healing and reparative, this eventually changes the patient's under-
developed affect-regulating structure, where the experience of attunement
and co-regulation eventually increases the capacity for modulation and self-
regulation. These mutative experiences help recalibrate the brain, allowing
for the brain to move out of automatic fear responses. This is because the
brain has developed a more regulated rhythm through the experience of
safety within the therapeutic relationship, thereby increasing the patient's
window of affect tolerance.

Ed Tronick and Claudia Gold's (2020) studies of infant/mother interactions reveal the importance of rupture and repair or disruption and repair
in the understanding of what comprises healthy attachment patterns. Their
early observations of mothers and infants in still-face experiments led them
to believe that synchronous and attuned interactions were what led to the
development of secure attachment patterns. However, after studying data
collected over decades of video-taped observations, they discovered that
typical infants and their caregivers were actually moving into states of
misattunement and repair on average *70 percent* of the time. Therefore, they
concluded, "The central lesson of decades of research following the original
still-face experiment is that this process of moving through mismatch to
repair is not only unavoidable but essential if relationships are to flourish
rather than stagnate or fall apart" (p. 39)."

Conversely, Tronick and Gold also observed that when there was little
opportunity for repair, infants did not make the same efforts to reengage
with the parent as contrasted with infant/parent dyads where repair was
consistently forthcoming. For infants whose mothers were preoccupied by
their own distress or mothers who behaved intrusively – for example,
hovering or repeatedly touching the infant even when the infant gives
signals of becoming overwhelmed, results in a learned passivity or a turning
inward. In turn this produces a shattered sense of self, a feeling of not being
seen or known. Tronick and Gold (2020) summarize by stating, "A person's physiological stress system is altered when the process of mismatch and
repair is derailed early in life. The experience lives in the body, and when
someone is stressed as an adult, the body may respond in ways shaped
by this early experience" (p. 217). When this happens in the therapeutic
relationship, we classify it as a transferential reenactment.

The discoveries in infant and child attachment research help us move
down the path of understanding intersubjective reality when working
with adult clients. The therapeutic process involves a series of continuous,

dynamic sequences of accommodation to rupture with the hope of repairing the connection, thus surviving breakdowns in mutual recognition. Developing the capacity to "recognize" the other means that both client and therapist must learn to tolerate certain degrees of stress as misattunements occur. In these moments, the illusion of the perfect other is shattered. However, it is by learning to stay with the stress of disappointed longings and processing the rupture together that reparation and co-regulation can occur.

Understanding this is foundational to working with transference and countertransference. When patients reveal their disappointment in the therapist without the therapist retaliating, this is a curative experience. When patients express negative emotions such as anger or mistrust and the therapist validates these feelings, this is a curative experience. When feelings of shame are exposed in the presence of the therapist and understood as a normal response to unhealthy situations in childhood, this can also become a curative experience.

Client Example

The following case vignette illustrates a situation where the patient experienced a rupture in her connection with the therapist. She was able to verbalize her disappointment the following week, and in that moment the therapist did not retaliate. Instead, she explored the source of the rupture, trying to understand it further. The outcome was a relational repair that not only increased trust in the alliance but increased the patient's sense of self agency.

Pt: *I was upset with you last week, and I've been meaning to talk to you about it.*
Th: *Yes?*
Pt: *I didn't like it when you said, "As you look ahead, given your diagnosis…" I know that we were talking about my difficulty making some pretty important life changes, and I know that I've struggled with this issue all of my life – I want to set limits, and I am also afraid to. But when you say, "What is most important to you as you look ahead given your diagnosis," it's not helpful. It actually makes me lose my focus and desire.*
Th: *Well, thank you for letting me know that. Was this difficult to bring this up with me?*
Pt: *Yes, it was, but I've been thinking about it all week, so I decided it was better to get it off my chest.*
Th: *I'm glad that you did.*
Pt: *Long pause … I mean, I'm well aware that my breast cancer has metastasized and it's likely that I won't stay in remission, but I don't want to think about it. I want to push it to the side.*
Th: *Ok. Can you help me understand how that is helpful to you?*

Pt: It helps me stay optimistic. It helps me stay in the present. None of us knows how much time we have left.

Th: So, pushing it aside actually helps you stay in the present? (pause) I'm wondering, what opens up for you when you stay in that space?

Pt: I can focus on my dance and my writing and practicing the violin. I actually get excited and look forward to these activities. But I know that I continue to struggle putting others first too much. I always take a back seat to other people's needs, and I take on too much with my job. I have difficulty saying no, but I do have to work, you know. I don't have the luxury of taking time off. And I'm tired all the time. I guess it's a mixed bag.

Th: A mixed bag?

Pt: Well, I can see that I swing back and forth – trying to create more space for myself while continuing to try to please others. And I know what you were trying to do when you said "given my diagnosis." You were wanting me not to slip into an old pattern. But I don't like it when you say it. I don't like to hear the words out loud.

Th: What would you rather have me say in these moments?

Pt: I don't know. Tell me I'm doing a good job, that I'm doing the best that I can, that these things are difficult for everybody, not just people with cancer looming over their heads. Please don't think I'm being critical of you right now.

Th: I didn't experience you as being critical or accusatory at all. How you just communicated all of this to me was very clear and very open. And now, as we've talked about it further, I can better see where you're coming from, how pushing it aside helps you stay focused and optimistic in the present, how that's actually an adaptive strategy for you, a way of making room for yourself without becoming overly fearful. So, we can find other ways to continue our conversation about this topic. What's most important is that you have expressed your disappointment with me, and we can talk it through together.

Pt: Thank you. You make it easier to practice speaking up. We've been doing therapy long enough that I do trust you not to retaliate. (Pause) You know, I'm well aware of my medical condition. Even though I push it aside, it's always there. I'm not in denial about it, and I realize I need to make some changes for myself. If not now, when?

Th: I guess that's where I was coming from last week, when I was referring to your diagnosis and what you wanted to do moving forward. I was trying to access some sense of urgency because that's what I thought you were trying to express to me, to find a way to talk about it together.

Pt: Yes, you're right. I was feeling more of a sense of urgency because I had just talked with my doctor. So, let's talk about how I can do that right now.

Questions for Consideration and Analysis

As you can see the therapist did not try to explain her intentions early in the exchange with her client.

1. From a transferential perspective, what opportunities did it give the client/therapist dyad to explore experientially?
2. Why do you think that the client *needed* to practice speaking up in order to create a reparative experience?
3. What further information was gained from allowing this exchange to unfold a bit longer?
4. What unexpressed longings may have been hidden within the client's exchange with the therapist that only surfaced when she experienced disappointment in her?
5. What fears might the client have held around expressing anger or disappointment directly?

After the client was able to express her disappointment without recrimination, he was able to additionally express what would have been more helpful and why it would have been more helpful. Letting the therapist know that she needed reassurance allowed him to express her anxiety while the therapist provided comfort in the present moment. After this part of the exchange had been completed, notice how the therapist continued to explore the possible negative transferential "parts" of the client's reactions when the client began to minimize or dismiss these parts. In this regard, the therapist attempted to access and normalize hidden aspects of both Q3 (the patient's longings for comfort) and Q4 (her disappointment and anger that in the past was forbidden to be expressed). Once they were able to explore both sides of this dilemma, the conflict was able to be held consciously and experientially between them. Therefore, at the end of this dialogic exchange, notice that the client was able to then go back to the more fearful side of the split on her own volition and acknowledge the importance of holding both parts of his present reality simultaneously. This internal shift was able to occur because the part of the client that had bristled over the direct reference to her cancer had been understood by the therapist, and her strategy for coping with her illness had been respected.

This client example illustrates the power of staying with the undercurrent of hidden transferential material in order that the patient's own reflective processes can become integrated and held consciously. One can see how shifting to historical material too early, before the transferential rupture was repaired in the present moment, might not have resulted in the same positive resolution. Engaging in the historical antecedents of reflexive patterns *after* a transferential rupture has been repaired experientially in the present moment can help to solidify the gains that occurred in the session.

Entrenched Transferential Enactments: Working with Metaphor and Humor to Break Through

One of the more difficult aspects of working with negatively entrenched transferential material centers on persistent dynamics that don't seem to shift despite repeated efforts on the part of the therapist to create safety and build a trusting alliance. Dan Siegel (1986) refers to these types of transferential sticking points occurring "when the patient unconsciously expects that the therapist, despite overt helpfulness and concern, will covertly exploit the patient for his or her own narcissistic gratification" (p. 72). Although the fear of exploitation remains unconscious, various forms of enactments can transpire that either create:

- a situation of mutual avoidance of the negative/fear-ridden self-states, resulting in a stalemate in the therapy where both therapist and client feel a combination of frustration and/or boredom,
- or the therapist may try to accommodate the patient's unconscious wishes, by overly attending to or overly identifying with the victim part of the split, resulting in increased dependency and/or increased demands of the therapist.

When therapeutic sticking points are difficult to break through, the therapist can engage in a dialogue where the issue of impasse is directly put on the table. The therapist can share from her own perspective what the relational exchange feels like, or where she feels caught in a bind. Or, the therapist can directly inquire how the process seems to be going from the patient's own perspective. This invitation opens a doorway to reflect upon and eventually expose underlying fears and/or disappointments coupled with the wish to possibly protect and/or punish the therapist. This process dialogue can be made to feel less threatening for the patient by introducing humor, play, or metaphor as a means of creating enough distance or neutral space in a way that hopefully allows for the normalization or neutralization of underlying fear and/or shame.

Metaphor takes the unconscious enactment of negative or fearful self-states, and turns them into symbolized form. Metaphor is a form of mentalization, where unformulated experience can be turned into symbolic organization in a way that a person can reflect on his/her own subjective meaning, affect, and intention (Fonagy et al., 2005). Metaphor coupled with play can often create a bridge of connection that allows nonconscious, forbidden material to be brought to the surface without the person becoming flooded or confused, thus being able to maintain a sense of personal control/self-coherence while remaining in connection with the therapist.

Donnel Stern (2010) states that for victims of trauma, the patient must be able to take in two vantage points at once, one that holds the traumatic experience and the other something else – a kind of reference that relates to the trauma but is nevertheless different. In this way the traumatic experience can be contextualized, and the traumatic memory can then become a part of the metaphor, an item in a category of associations that has become more neutralized. Only when the patient is able to know the experience in this way can the interpersonal field feel emotionally safe and responsive enough (p. 137). Stern's description of how metaphor can be used to turn the interpersonal field into an experience that can feel safe and responsive enough is illustrated through the following client example.

Client Example One

This case illustration reveals a persistent, almost suffocating dynamic where the client would talk incessantly from the moment she came into the session. The therapist described the experience as the patient having no punctuation in her thought, no pause in the monologue. Every sentence ended with "and" followed by a new piece of information. This pattern and experience of being with the client lasted for months. If the therapist interrupted the flow of the patient's dialogue, it was as if her presence or her comment couldn't penetrate the patient's "wall of words." After some period of time, the therapist posed this comment, *"I have a question for you. I'm wondering how it's going for you in here because I know you come here for support and help, but I'm also noticing that you're not hearing much from me, and you're not requesting much from me." "Is that enough for you? How is that for you?"* The patient initially responded by saying that yes, it was enough explaining that she just needed to be heard. The therapist reported that at that time the patient didn't seem to be interested in looking into her behavior as a pattern or a problematic dynamic that repeated every session.

Progression

The next time the therapist decided to bring up a reflective comment was in relation to the patient's anxiety. The therapist reported that every time she was about to speak, the patient would look away, or she would just begin to talk over the therapist. Even though the patient knew on some level that the therapist had something to say, she was actively, although not consciously, seeming to push the therapist away. At one point when the theme of anxiety was at the forefront of several sessions, the therapist decided to start the session with some grounding, breathing, and centering techniques. The therapist stated that the patient seemed to have a very difficult time settling down with the centering exercises. She continued to exhibit physical agitation and interrupted the breathing exercises with questions or comments.

At that point, the therapist made another reflective comment saying, *"Would you like to hear what I'm seeing as we try to do this exercise together, what you look like from the outside? (Pause) You look like a hummingbird. You know how hummingbirds are constantly moving? It's a part of their nature."* The patient liked that image, and the therapist used a sense of playfulness by saying, "*I don't know what it feels like to you, but it looks like your hummingbird is working very hard right now.*" The patient laughed and said, "*I love hummingbirds.*"

Clearly, this metaphor worked to create a sense of relational safety which seemed to break the reflexive pattern of self-protection. It also seemed to register with the patient in a place that felt descriptively true while also being congruent with her self-image. By offering this metaphor, it was the first time that the patient was able to accept a reflective comment from the therapist. She seemed to be able to take the comment in, incorporating it into her identity in a way that both therapist and patient could acknowledge together.

Over the course of several sessions the therapist began to introduce other reflective comments, building upon this metaphor. One comment she made was, "*The hummingbird has to keep moving all the time, and I'm wondering what would happen if the hummingbird landed. I'm wondering if we could consider that together, talk about what might happen if she landed.*"

Later, the therapist was able to say, "*It feels rude for me to interrupt you, but I'm wondering if I could have your permission to interrupt you in the service of both of us gaining some understanding as to why it is necessary for the hummingbird to work so hard. From where I sit, it's as if you have to do all of the work in here all by yourself.*"

The patient agreed to allow the therapist to interrupt. Asking permission to interrupt gave the patient a sense of personal control. She could choose whether to stop herself or let the therapist know she needed to keep talking. Eventually, the patient began to catch herself in the middle of a long explanation and state, "*I'm doing it again, aren't I?*" The patient's growing capacity to self-reflect was a way for her to metabolize her hovering, ever-present anxiety. Over time the therapist and patient could look at the feeling of anxiety and the image of the hummingbird as a positive and adaptive strategy to early traumatic memories. They were able to get in touch with what the patient was trying to prevent, her fear of a rupture in their relational connection. Accessing this consciously allowed for a breakthrough in the enactment.

The Therapist's Analysis and Reflections

The therapist reported that this patient's early life was filled with chronic attachment failures where the patient experienced a sense of complete isolation when she was in need of comfort coupled with parents who were harsh and overly controlling. The therapist believed that the patient's attempt to fill the session with her own talk was an unconscious attempt to guard against further relational disappointment. Upon reflection, the therapist stated, "*What was wonderful about this case was that I found a way to interrupt this unconscious enactment with metaphor and with humor. Eventually, we were able to access her underlying fears. When she was able to become trusting enough* to let me engage with her more directly, she was then able to become curious about the dynamic that had been created between us in the first months of therapy. Eventually she was able to find the words to say, 'Maybe I'm afraid you're going to say the wrong thing'."

From there, the therapist reported that they were able to explore what might happen if she did say the wrong thing. "*My patient feared that if I said anything and it was the wrong thing, it might have created a sense of such profound disappointment that it would shatter the fragile, positive connection we had established. Essentially, she feared that she would be unable to prevent experiencing the sense of abandonment again and the rage that she might direct at me if I said the wrong thing. She said that she counted on me and didn't want to lose me.*"

The image of the hummingbird seemed to create a bridge, a safe way to allow hidden feelings to come to the surface. It increased the patient's capacity for flexibility and elasticity. By using the positive association to the metaphor, she could laugh about her own behavior; she could experience it without feeling ashamed. She then began to feel that she had more room to interact differently; she felt that she now had a choice. She could be the hummingbird, but she also didn't have to be the hummingbird in flight. Then, if the therapist would interrupt her, the patient felt that she had the capacity to make a choice, rather than being under the dominion of a controlling other. This patient could either stop talking and let her therapist engage with her, or she could say "*No, I really need to finish this story. I don't want you to talk right now.*" In that way the patient could experience the freedom of moving back into a familiar protective space when she needed to, and the therapist allowed enough permission and flexibility that the patient felt the freedom of her own choices.

When asked about any counter-transferential reactions, the therapist stated that it was initially challenging to sit in the room and feel that you have something to offer but weren't given any opportunity to intervene. She stated, "*I was able to experience her distress, experience my own wish to contribute and be helpful, but I felt continually thwarted. I also felt stuck. I knew that I had to proceed slowly. So, I initially took her at her word and gave her the space to talk and not be interrupted. I knew on some level that she needed to have an actual experience with another where she could fill the space with her own presence without someone taking over or overpowering her. There were literally countless sessions where I could barely say two words. On one level, I felt silenced, and that was challenging for me. Then I realized this is what must have happened to her as a child. I knew she had an extremely domineering father. I didn't have more details other than that, but I was able to glean what it must have felt like growing up with him simply by sitting in those initial sessions of our work together. Once I figured this out, it took a while for me to hold this construct, to stay with her, but to try to engage with her in a way that would be productive.*"

In my debrief with the therapist, I asked her how the metaphor of the hummingbird came to mind because it seemed to be such a constructive and accurate experiential description of what was happening in the room.

The therapist responded by saying that all she could imagine was that there was so much going on right brain to right brain. *"It just seemed that energetically there was enough softness that was being created between us over time, that eventually I sensed that there was an opening, or maybe I came to understanding so deeply what she was communicating viscerally that the metaphor just popped into my mind. When I shared the image of the hummingbird, it was the first time she stopped talking, and she seemed genuinely interested in connecting."*

This client example is a clear illustration of how metaphor can translate pre-symbolic memory into an organizing schematic that can apply language and positive associations as a bridge for self-reflection. Even though this enactment reflected learned behaviors that were acquired in her early dominant-submissive relationship with her father, a neutral metaphor was able to capture the relational dynamic experienced between the therapist and patient while highlighting the adaptive aspects of preserving self in relationship. Rather than raising into consciousness the unknown parts of the self that may unconsciously mimic the aggressor's behavior, metaphor can be a benign way of bridging this gap.

Client Example Two

Metaphor can also be a communication from the patient to the therapist. Often times the patient's transferential feelings are conveyed through dreams, acting as a metaphor that capture complex relational dynamics in symbolic form. In this client example Margaret, a long-term patient, had been making steady progress in her treatment with Dr. K. Their initial work involved a repeated relational enactment where Margaret assumed a state of passive dependence coupled with repeated boundary testing of Dr. K. where she demanded that he prove his caring for her by giving her special privileges or sharing personal information about himself. At one point during her treatment the patient experienced a relational rupture when Dr. K forgot an important detail from a traumatic episode with her mother. With Dr. K's apology, it appeared that the playing field had leveled, and a shift gradually occur in their relationship as Margaret began to display increased signs of autonomy. Dr. K's encouragement and praise of her progress also helped Margaret demonstrate signs of self-agency in the outside world where she no longer drifted from part-time waitressing jobs but was able to apply her undergraduate degree to procure a full-time position at a biotech company.

Then an incident occurred that created a set-back for Margaret. While in the waiting room prior to a session, she overheard Dr. K. speaking in an animated fashion to another patient. She immediately felt that Dr. K. was more comfortable with this patient, and that working with Margaret was far less satisfying. At this point Margaret's longing that she could be "the special one" got shattered. During that session, Dr. K. sensed that something had occurred because Margaret was withdrawn, at a loss for words. In their next session, Margaret was able to articulate what had happened in the waiting room and explained that she felt herself detaching from the connection with Dr. K. in that moment. Remarkably, she was able to access these feelings by remembering a dream she had had the night before. *"I had a dream where you were on the dock, and I was in a boat. You were throwing me a line, but I felt that you were also letting me drift away from the dock on my own. The rope you were holding was getting longer and longer as I moved further away from the dock. You were letting me go, and I wasn't ready. I remember hearing myself thinking that I had lost the feeling of us in connection. There is no more of us working together."*

Remarkably, what Margaret was able to access this dream metaphor to describe to Dr. K. the visual and felt sense of their relational state after she felt the disappointment and rupture in the waiting room. Here is where the therapist can use the metaphor to provide real reassurance of the relational connection to help create a reparative experience. In this instance Dr. K. built upon the metaphor by saying, *"You are helping me understand your situation. You don't want me to leave you in that boat alone, too soon."* Two simple sentences that convey, I hear you, I understand the complexity of your situation, and I'm not going to ask you to leave therapy prematurely.

Upon hearing this reassurance, Margaret was then able to communicate to him that although she's aware that she's made progress in therapy, she still didn't have "a motor," she still didn't have all the tools she needed, and that meant she is still in peril. Once these fears were verbalized, Margaret was able to relax and feel reconnected. Again, the power of metaphor can help translate unarticulated feeling states into a dream experience that can capture the essence of a relational rupture or a buried unrequited longing.

Understanding Loyalty Contracts as a Transferential Enactment

In Chapter Five you were introduced to the concept of loyalty contracts as a means of reenacting dysfunctional relational patterns in present-day relationships. These patterns will eventually manifest in transferential and counter-transferential communications. Simply put, one way to understand transferential enactments is through articulating the patient's learned loyalty contract. Developing a clearer grasp of the parental messages that were conveyed through early loyalty contracts can be accessed through your own counter-transferential responses to the patient.

Unfair loyalty contracts demand a quid pro quo interaction where the child is not seen and valued for their unique selves; rather the relationship is based on the parent's narcissistic wishes or need to dominate and control the child. Therefore, the dominant/subordinate position will often play out transferentially through the reenactment of the loyalty contract. At times the patient will play the subservient role and either enact a request for rescue or salvation, or the patient may enact a response of withholding and mistrust, fearing that the therapist will eventually become the dominant, controlling other. Conversely, the therapist may feel on the receiving end of the victim position in a reenactment of a dominant/submissive loyalty contract. At these times, the therapist may feel that s/he can't do anything right, or the client may exert pressure, making demands for atonement and/or retribution if disappointed by the relationship. In these transferential/counter-transferential situations, a therapist can often feel lost, without a clear picture of which side of the enactment is at play at any given moment. This is when giving language to what is being expressed in terms of the loyal contract demands can be a useful exercise in the service of breaking through a transferential/counter-transferential impasse.

Client Example

In the following client example, the therapist began to feel an increasing amount of irritability and frustration toward her patient after working with her for approximately six months. Although she initially experienced the client as quite likeable, she didn't quite understand her growing frustration. The therapist described the client as attractive, intelligent, hard-working, and personally responsible, almost to a fault. The therapist reported, however, that she had begun to observe a repeated cycle where the patient would drive herself to exhaustion with work projects, followed by periods of mental and physical collapse where she had to take short breaks from work, only to repeat the cycle once she physically recovered. Although the therapist tried to direct the client's attention to the cost of this pattern, the client was to acknowledge this intellectually, but the behavior continued to manifest.

Background: This is a young Asian woman in her early thirties who was adopted by a white family in Southern California. Parents provided basic necessities such as shelter and a quality education, but the expectation from the family was that the patient needed to be self-reliant as well as assuming the role of caretaker for her younger siblings. She reported that she loved her parents, but they never allowed her to express herself; they didn't believe in crying or showing emotions. There was an older brother in her house, not her biological brother, who was also adopted and had addiction and anger issues. The patient reported that he was very unpredictable and exhibited scary behaviors. He was combative toward her parents and he "did sexual things" to her when she was between 4 and 6 years old. She never told her parents because she did not want to upset them.

The patient had one psychiatric hospitalization for 8 days for suicidal ideation and one suicide attempt at age 16, where she tried to hang herself. The patient reports a history of depression and anxiety since she was in high school, and reports being diagnosed with PTSD. Currently, the patient is estranged from her three siblings and adopted father. The details of this alienation are unclear, and the patient is not forthcoming with this information.

She is currently in a committed, live-in relationship. She expects her boyfriend and friends to understand her and support her, although she often resists their efforts to intervene and help. Her trust in others is tentative. She actively questions her current relationship, "He does not believe in my mental health concerns or need for medication, and he thinks my symptoms aren't real." The therapist reported that the patient's expectation of mutuality and fairness in relationships appeared to be a bit confused. She is living with her boyfriend, expects him to tolerate her dramatic withdrawals, and she shows great reluctance to do things that might help her own situation. In addition, she appears to offer little affection or attention to the boyfriend in return.

The patient entered treatment because of exhaustion following an emotional breakdown at work. During these episodes the patient reported losing track of time and feeling "unreal." In session, she would often dissociate when asked questions about her feelings of "just wanting to collapse." Nor could she articulate what would be of help to get her back on her feet. During the course of therapy, the therapist felt that the patient had very little belief that anything would get better regardless of what she did or what anyone else might do for her. Any gentle suggestion of things she might do differently were immediately rejected. At these moments she would either express some impatience with the therapist, and if pressed, she would appear to dissociate. The patient self-disclosed that she "checks-out" (dissociates) when she experiences anything that triggers memories of past trauma or when she pushes herself to work hard at school to get things done. A typical pattern for her is to work extremely hard on a project or a clinical rotation and once it's done, to sleep for days which she describes as both peaceful and a form of dissociation.

During a consultation session the therapist confessed that she was feeling stuck and didn't know how to make any inroads into what felt like a wall of avoidance when feelings came close to the surface. The therapist admitted that she was getting frustrated with the patient's complaints because "*It always felt that there was an entitled edge to them.*" Our consultation group was able to break through some of her counter transferential reactions to the patient by focusing on the transference/counter-transference enactment through the lens of understanding the patient's early loyalty contract.

We were able to frame the loyalty contract from two points of view, one from the position of being the victim who was on the receiving end of trauma, and the other from the position of either the entitled or abusive aggressor. We articulated the loyal contract based on the patient's behaviors and underlying expectations of self and other that the therapist was able to observe during the course of their work together. We first framed the enactment from the vantage-point of the victim and tried to articulate the underlying wish contained within the enactment. In doing so, the loyalty contract sounded like this:

> *If I tell you how much I'm suffering, will you pay attention to me and take care of me? You know, nobody took care of me in the past, so you really need to prove to me that you won't let me down, because I can't be disappointed one more time. You see, I'm doing my part, I take care of others, I'm doing the best I can, now you do the same for me.*
>
> *But if you do reach out and try to help, I can't really accept it because secretly I don't feel worthy to be taken care of; I don't feel worthy to even be alive. My birth mother let me go; so that must mean I'm not worth much. How can I ever trust that anyone would be any different Look, my own mother gave me away and my parents couldn't protect me from my brother who raped me.*
>
> *You see, I secretly believe that no one can help, but damn it, I'm really tired of trying to do this by myself.*

The articulation of the loyalty contract from the point of view of the victim illustrates how the wish for rescue stays alive. However, the patient guards herself against receiving help for fear of disappointment or further abuse. In an unconscious way, it is also a way that she is able maintain a connection - to remain loyal to her parents and her birth mother. However, this represents only one half of the conflict contained within the transferential enactment. The "not me" part of the self has absorbed the demanding position that the parents placed on her as a child and the brutal treatment she received from her brother. This demanding part of the enactment is alive and is projected onto important others in the form of the patient's high expectation.

Therefore, if we were to reverse the enacted communication from that of helpless victim (the done to position) to the voice of the dominant parent, brother/aggressor (the doer position), the therapist has a clearer picture of the pressure she feels counter-transferentially. By giving language to what must have been the aggressor's demands, the therapist could then feel what it must have felt like being on the receiving end of the loyalty contract. The articulation of the demand contained within the split-off part of the communication/enactment might sound like this:

> *"Because I sacrificed myself and kept my mouth shut, now you must take care of me and not complain! You can't get frustrated or tell me to pull myself together because I'm paying you for this. If you disappoint me or fall short, I get to distance from you and criticize you.*
>
> *And you can't ask me to do anything to take care of myself. If you do try to make me responsible, I will collapse into dissociative oblivion, and you can't challenge me on that because that's how I find relief. You see, I don't have to be*

held accountable. Nobody ever held my birth mother or my brother accountable. Now it's my turn. What I really need is to find the perfect caretaker. Then all of my sacrifice will have been worth it."

Once the loyalty contract is verbalized from the vantage-point of an unconscious deeply entrenched demand, the therapist was able to make sense out of her counter-transferential frustration. She was also able to regain her compassion for the unrequited longings that we never met by this adopted young girl. Feelings were forbidden in her family of origin, therefore, they needed to be split-off and remained as unformulated experience. Once regaining this clarity, the therapist was able to articulate what she imagined her patient was trying to communicate on a deeper, visceral level. She expressed it in these words.

> *"You need to understand, the only way I know of experiencing any kind of self-worth comes from losing myself in work or sacrificing for others. I don't have anything else to organize my identity, and if I stop, I won't know who I am. So, we're not going to go there. I can't talk about it because I don't have the words. There's nothing there. That's when I disappear."*

Once the therapist was able to articulate the reason for the patient's overdetermined efforts at maintaining self-coherence, she was then able to see that she needed to help the patient build a bridge, give her verbal structures that she might be able to hold onto. The consultation group began to brainstorm as to what might be useful reflections.

- One suggestion was that the therapist could begin to mirror to the patient parts of herself that were either minimized or not known. By reflecting these undervalued or unknown parts of herself back to the patient, the patient might gradually begin to broaden her definition of "the good me" in relation to others.
- Another suggestion was to point out the extremes in the patient's thinking and behavior – she was either all-sacrificing or in total collapse. By introducing decision-making choices that included self-care and limit-setting with other people's expectations could help the patient begin to self-differentiate while maintaining a relational connection to others.
- A third suggestion was to anticipate what it might feel like to move toward having less perfectionistic expectations of herself and/or others. Would she feel let down, disappointed? Was this a way of protecting herself from feeling her anger, her grief? Listening for opportunities to enter into this dialogue allowed the therapist see where their work was headed.
- A fourth suggestion was to have the therapist give actual language to the loyalty contract dilemma. The therapist could begin by naming the parts of her unconscious behavioral enactments more directly. For

example, she might say, *"I can see that you work so hard, and there is clearly such a payoff. You help so many people, and I'm sure it gives you an enormous amount of satisfaction. It also allows you to stay out of your head when difficult feelings sometimes come up. But we've also talked about how this exhausts you. Are you aware of these conflicting parts of yourself?"* Naming these parts aloud is how the therapist might begin to speak to the splits, so that the unknown parts are able to be acknowledged along with the parts that are more known or syntonic.

- Finally, the therapist could focus on the relationship with her live-in partner. Asking for specific examples of what she felt she had a right to expect from her relationship may set the stage for increasing the patient's capacity for self-reflection as well as raising into conscious awareness her pattern of reactivity and/or retaliation whenever she experiences disappointment. As a start, the therapist might ask, *"What were you hoping he would have done that would have felt better to you?"* *"How might you share your disappointment with him without shutting down or pulling away?"* *"What do you tell yourself it means when he falls short?"*

Focusing on specific questions allows the therapist to access entry points into the patient's hidden assumptions and reactions. Eventually, speaking with this level of specificity helps the unrequited wishes and longings come to the surface.

The importance of articulating transferential dilemmas using the framework of *learned loyalty contracts* can often help therapists hold more of the complexity of the enactment in conscious awareness. Once the multiple dimensions of an enactment become clear to therapists, they can regain their balance and shift into a position of "rhythmic third" by using countertransferential feelings to assist in regaining a sense of connection, by using a light touch, saying something clinically relevant but with a bit of humor to maintain connectivity. Finally, when the therapist is able to frame enactments through the lens of learned loyalty contracts, it generally helps the patient connect present longings and fears to their own historical experience, which in turn helps to interrupt repeated patterns and disentangle the past from the present.

Summary

Understanding the relationship between transference and countertransference is at the heart of all relationally based psychotherapies. It is in the intersubjective space created within the therapeutic relationship where unresolved fears, longings, and relational assumptions emerge. It is in this same intersubjective space that new experiences of safety and connection have the healing power to replace reflexive reactions and limiting relational assumptions. Working with transference and countertransference is the arena in which enactments are brought into conscious awareness, the successful resolution of which will eventually reshape the client's narrative of self and self in relationship.

Learned loyalty contracts determine attachment patterns that are later reenacted in adulthood through transferential projections onto significant others as well as the therapist. These repeating patterns represent unresolved wishes or fears, and they can be identified as such when patients appear to be unable to learn from mistakes and/or experience similar disappointments in relationships across various contexts. The majority of symptoms that clients present upon entering therapy provide a window into understanding how early attachment failures resulted in acts of over-compensation or lack of self-care. In fact, many times symptoms can be viewed as a physiological manifestation of an enactment, the body's way of giving us clues as to what went wrong, how the patient has tried to cope, and what needs our attention so that repair and balance can occur.

Before repair can happen, questions that help access the meaning of relational enactments need to be answered, questions such as:

- What is the function of this symptom or this enactment?
- What are the underlying wishes or longings that are contained within the enactment?
- Is there a double bind that the patient is placing on the therapist due to an underlying assumption that the patient is making?
- How does the enactment serve as a protection against feelings of shame or feelings of vulnerability?
- How is the issue of safety or lack of safety being enacted?

Hopefully, this chapter has helped address these questions as well as offering examples of how to access what patients are trying to communicate through actions or enactments that have yet to assume conscious, articulated form.

Transferential enactments *always* telegraph information to the therapist. What is split off or dissociated eventually becomes enacted in the transference. Therapists register these split-off parts of the patient's psyche both consciously, in the form of their clinical observations and reflections, as well as unconsciously, through their corresponding counter-transferential feelings and responses. Because transference is the portal that connects prior wounds to present-day enactments, working with transference in the unfolding present also enables the therapist to see how early attachment injuries (the rules contained in learned loyalty contracts) manifest in relationship.

The aim of any transferential dialogic exchange is to open a doorway to engage the client's curiosity as to new possibilities for connection. This is done by providing reassurance, correcting misunderstandings, or giving permission for negative reactions to be present without the patient having to experience retaliation on the part of the therapist. It is only when the therapist treats the patient differently than s/he expects that the patient can then experience a new way of being in relationship with another. Over time, the accumulation of repeated positive experiences within the context of the therapeutic relationship, including the successful resolution of ruptures of attunement, gives our patients an opportunity to challenge their learned, habituated assumptions. It is through the processing and reprocessing of enactments that a more benign experience of being in relationship slowly becomes internalized as past relational failures gradually become ameliorated by successful, present-day relational exchanges.

As Donnel Stern (2009) most eloquently summarizes, "Even in the absence of others, we learn about ourselves by imaginatively listening to our own thoughts through the ears of the other. At the beginning of life, we need a witness to become a self. Later, patients listen to themselves as they imagine their analysts hear them, and in this way create new narrative freedom. The resolution of enactments is crucial in psychoanalytic treatment, not only because it expands the boundaries of the self, but also because it reinstitutes and broadens the range within which patient and analyst can witness one another's experience. Narrative is not the outcome of the analyst's objective interpretations, but an emergent, co-constructed, unbidden outcome of clinical process" (p. 701).

It takes a *clear* witness for a person to become an authentically integrated self, something our patients never experienced when they were young. Instead, they come to us bearing the damage that was done to them by the faulty witnessing of others. They enter into therapy hoping that we will be able to make a difference but expecting that we will somehow inflict damage upon them just the same. This hidden fear/expectation is perhaps one of the most under-examined dynamics that eventually becomes a part of every therapeutic engagement. This is why understanding and working with transferential enactments has become the backbone of doing transformative therapeutic work. For our patients so much of who they fully are has remained unwitnessed, or worse, has been shamed and sequestered into split off parts of the self that remain unknown or unknowable.

As we gain comfort and confidence with navigating the transferential/counter-transferential space of therapeutic engagement, this becomes a powerful mirror that allows our patients to be seen through the eyes and ears of another. We can see parts of them that represent their gifts and talents, precious parts of the self that were undervalued or went unacknowledged by their caregivers. We also see the parts of our patients that are out of balance, driven by over-determined efforts to prove that they are worthy or loveable. We eventually experience the unacknowledged parts of our patients, where feelings of terror or shame remain sequestered in self-states that had to be split off and remain unknowable.

Our patients are also able to see and eventually challenge parts of us that become intertwined in the relational mix, sorted out through the ongoing dance of rupture and repair. Adjusting our perspective to hold both the field and ground of relational intersubjectivity requires a delicate touch, filled with compassionate reflection and an internal steadiness to help us weather the therapeutic storms. This process forces us to become humble learners as we slowly master the skills necessary to hold the complexity and fragility of human interaction. This is how the disavowed parts of the self can gradually be integrated into an expanding sense of self-acceptance and possibility, thus creating a new narrative freedom.

References

Balint, M. (1968). *The basic fault*. Tavistock.

Benjamin, J. (2018). *Beyond doer and done to: Recognition theory, intersubjectivity and the third*. Routledge.

Benjamin, J. (2019). Pre-Conference lecture - beyond 'doer and done to: Putting the theory of "the third" into clinical practice*. Psychodynamic Psychotherapy 2019, The Lawrence E. Lifon, MD, Psychotherapy Conference.

Black, M. (2003) Enactment: Analytic musings on energy, language, and personal growth. *Psychoanalytic Dialogues, 13*(5), 633–635.

Botella, C., & Botella, S. (2005). *The work of psychic figurability*. Brunner/Routledge.

Bollas, C. (2009). *The infinite question*. Routledge.

Brickman, C. (2018). *Race in psychoanalysis: Aboriginal populations in the mind*. Routledge.

Bromberg, P. M. (1998). *Standing in the spaces: Essays on clinical process, trauma and dissociation*. Analytic Press.

Brown, J. (2017). *Counseling diversity in context*. University of Toronto Press.

Brown, J. (2019). *Anti-oppressive counseling and psychotherapy: Action for personal and social change*. Routledge.

Cozolino, L. (2002). *The neuroscience of psychotherapy: Building and rebuilding the human brain*. W.W. Norton & Company.

Cozolino, L. (2006). *The neuroscience of human relationships: Attachment and the developing social brain*. W.W. Norton & Company.

Danielian, J., & Gianotti, P. (2012). *Listening with purpose: Entry points into shame and narcissistic vulnerability*. Routledge.

Ferenczi, S. (1919). Contra-indications to the "active" psycho-analytical technique. In J. Rickman (Ed.) & J. Suttie (Trans.), *Further contributions to the theory and technique of psycho-analysis* (pp. 189–197). Boni and Liveright.

Fisher, J. (2021). *Transforming the living legacy of trauma: A workbook for survivors and therapists*. PESI Publishing & Media.

Fonagy, P., Greely, G., Jurist, E. L., & Targer, M. (2005). *Affect regulation, mentalization, and the development of the self*. Other Press.

Greenson, R. R. (1968). *The technique and practice of psychoanalysis: Volume 1*. Generic.

Ginot, E. (2007). Intersubjectivity and neuroscience: Understanding enactments and their therapeutic significance with emerging paradigms. *Psychoanalytic Psychology, 24*, 317–332.

Ginot, E. (2009). The empathic power of enactments: The link between neuropsychological processes and an expanded definition of empathy. *Psychoanalytic Psychology, 26*(3), 290–309.

Grossmark, R. (2016). Psychoanalytic companioning. *Psychoanalytic Dialogues, 26*(6), 698–712.

Grossmark, R. (2018). *The unobtrusive relational analyst: Explorations in psychoanalytic companioning.* Routledge.

Howell, E. F. (2005). *The dissociative mind.* Routledge: Taylor & Francis Group

Lanius. U. F., Paulsen, S. L., & Corrigan, F. M. (2014). *Neurobiology and treatment of traumatic dissociation: Toward an embodied self.* Springer Publishing Company.

Leary, K. (2000). Racial enactments in dynamic treatment. *Psychoanalytic Dialogues, 10*(4), 639–653.

Long, C., Matee, H., Jwili, O., & Vilakazi, Z. (2020). *Psychoanalytic Dialogues, 30,* 698–715. Routledge.

Lyons-Ruth, K. (1999). The two-person unconscious: Intersubjective dialogue, enactive relational representation, and the emergence of new forms of relational organization. *Psychoanalytic Inquiry, 19*(4), 576–617.

Maroda, K. J. (2020). Deconstructing enactment. *Psychoanalytic Psychology, 37*(1), 8–17. https://doi.org/10.1037/pap0000282.

Myers, V. (2011). *Moving diversity forward: How to go from well-meaning to well-doing.* Chicago: American Bar Association Center for Racial and Ethnic Diversity General Practice, Solo & Small Firm Division.

Schore, A. N. (2012). *The science of the art of psychotherapy.* W. W Norton & Company.

Siegel, D. (1986). Dissociation, double binds, and post-traumatic stress in multiple personality disorder. In B. G. Braun (Ed.), *Treatment of Multiple Personality Disorder.* American Psychiatric Press.

Stern, D.B. (2009). Partners in thought: A clinical process theory of narrative. *Psychoanalytic Quarterly, 78,* 701–731.

Stern, D. B. (2010). *Partners in thought: Working with unformulated experience, dissociation, and enactment.* Routledge.

Stern, D. B. (2015). *Relational freedom: Emergent properties of the relational field.* Routledge.

Stolorow, R. D. (2013). Intersubjective-systems theory: A phenomenological-contextualist psychoanalytic perspective. *Psychoanalytic Dialogues, 23,* 383–389. Routledge: Taylor Francis Group.

Tronick, E., & Gold, C. M. (2020). *The power of discord: Why the ups and downs of relationships are the secret to building intimacy, resilience, and trust.* Little, Brown Spark.

van der Kolk, B. (2015). *The body keeps the score: Brain, mind, and body in the healing of trauma.* Penguin Books.

Wallin, D. J. (2007). *Attachment in psychotherapy.* Guilford Press.

Winnicott, D. W. (1951). Transitional objects and transitional phenomena. In *Through paediatrics to psychoanalysis* (pp. 229–242). Basic Books.

Winnicott, D. W. (1965). *The maturational processes and the facilitating environment: Studies in the theory of emotional development.* Hogarth Press and the Institute of Psychoanalysis.

Zetzel, E. R. (1970). *The capacity for emotional growth.* The International Psychoanalytical Library, Khan, M. R. (Ed.). The Hogarth Press.

Index

Note that the italicized "*f*" after a page number refers to a figure.

A
Adler, A. 22
affect dysregulation 1
affective language 6
affective schemas 83
Ainsworth, M. D. S. 6
Akhtar, S. 82
Alexander, F. 7
Allport, G. W. 22
American Psychological Association
   (APA) 6, 61
anxiety 32
Aron, L. 147
assessment tools 3
attachment theory 3, 6; attachment needs
   as hard-wired 8; failures result in under-
   developed sense of self 28; grounding in
   as unifying principle of psychodynamic
   practice 8; idealized figures 33;
   identification of conditions and factors
   for secure attachment 6; infant and
   child in 205–206; insecure attachments
   shown in Four Quadrant Model 26,
   27–28; loss of idealized objects 33;
   over-reliance on figures of attachment
   33; shift to regulation theory 88;
   tenuous parental attachment styles 147;
   trauma and 204
Atwood, G. E. 147
autistic-like states 178–179
Ayoub, C. 158, 161

B
Balint, M. 182, 189
Beebe, B. 6, 13, 58
behavioral psychopathology 1
Bell, S. M. 6

Bellak, L. 22
Benjamin, J. 57–58, 143, 189, 192, 198, 199
Benjamin, L. S. 82
Bion, W. R. 32
Black, M. J. 32, 193
blame 52
Bollas, C. 189
borderline assessment category 82
Boston Change Process Study Group 156
Bowlby, J. 6
Brickman, C. 192
British Middle Group 189
Bromberg, P. 6, 157, 159, 185, 190
Brown, J. 192
Bucci, W. 81, 83, 185

C
Carlson, E. 158
case conceptualization 5, 16; the art of
   79–80; complexity of 81; Four
   Quadrant Model in 10, 16
caste systems 59–60
change based on lived experience 12
character formation organizing schemas
   143–144; as base for self 39; direct
   impact of on treatments 43; dominant
   trends in 40–41; movement against
   people trend 42, 44–45; movement
   away people trend 42, 45; movement
   toward people trend 41, 43–44
Chu, James 157
clinical application 3
clinical styles 24
cognitive behavioral strategies 2; as major
   orientation in psychotherapy 7
cognitive flexibility 22
collective social construction 59–60

compassionate attitude 81
compliant or over-attached self-effacing solution 41–42, 43–44; compulsivity behind 41
component parts of psyche 3
Confusion of Tongues Between Adults and the Child (Ferenczi) 51
Cordoba, A. I. 22
countertransference 8, 17–18, 188, 189, 206
counter-transferential experience 55–57; as ongoing exchange between therapist and patient 57
Cozolino, L. 204
Crastnopol, M. 147, 150, 156
The Crown (tv series) 49
Csikszentmihalyi, M. 159
cultural marginalization 89–90
cultural norms 8
Cyr, C. 6

D

Danielian, J. 9, 14, 22, 39, 41, 46, 111, 143, 159, 162, 188
Deci, E. L. 46
defense-driven model of psychic organization 15
defense mechanisms 9, 23; measurement of adaptive *vs.* maladaptive 87; measurement of rigidity of patient's 37; splitting 17, 40
de-idealization process 33–34; alters views of the self 33
DeRosis, L. 143
developmental phases 32
developmental trauma 38–39
DeYoung, P. 157, 162
diagnostic tools 23–24
dialogic process: importance of slowing down 10–11; transference and counter transference in 18
differentiation 143
dissociation model 154–155; barrier between self-states from 162–163; compartmentalization of information and affect function 159; critical aspects of emotional development 154–155; damages from early childhood traumas 157–158; as defence against state of identity 157; definition 157; dividing attention into streams of consciousness function 158–159; early emotional development incorporated into

154–155; functions of 158–160; healthy as flow experience 159; identification and distancing of self function 159; as neurologically based involuntary reflex 155; non-existence of *me* in 176–177; of self-states 154, 160–161; splitting as form of 156–157; traumatic dissociation 160
dissociative episodes 6
Dissociative Experiences Scale 158
dissociative self-states 157–158
domination 57, 59
double bind messages 61–65
Dutra, L. 6
duty 49
dynamic formulation 3
dynamic interaction between patient and therapist 5

E

early parent–infant interaction 6
ego psychologists 32
ego strengths 22
Elliott, R. 83
Emotion Focused Therapy (EFT) 75, 82
Erickson, E. H. 22, 32
Eurocentrism 89–90
evolving lifespan model of psychic organization 15
evolving self 3
expansive solution: the appeal of mastery 42, 44–45; compulsivity behind 42
explicit information processing 12, 13
expressive therapy 82

F

Fairbairn, W. R. D. 22, 32
familial/cultural expectations as shapers of identity 49
Ferenczi, S. 7, 51, 189
Ferro, A. 178, 179
figure, concept of 8
Fischer, K. W. 158, 161
Fisher, J. 204
Fonagy, P. 209
Four Quadrant Model 9, 10, 15; as an assessment tool 92–98, 93*f;* in case conceptualization 16, 89–92; compared to healthy self-actualizing model 25*f*, 35, 36*f;* connects defense mechanisms 10; definition of quadrants in 27, 30–31; distinction between conscious *vs.* dissociative process in 26; early

attachment failures shown by 26, 27–28; entry points in 114–117, 119–121; as graphic of learned defence mechanisms 9; for graphic of psychic injury 22–23; as picture of personality organization 161–162, 162*f*; psychodynamic template for 98–102; qualities of narcissistic overcompensation in 29–31, 30*f*; as safety net 24; splitting and 17; structural design of 24–26; as teaching tool 23; as tightly woven construction of interconnecting parts 31; uses in assessment and treatment 37–38
fractionation 161
Frank, R. 6
Frederickson, B. L. 22
French, T. M. 7
Freud, S. 7, 32
Friedman, R. S. 82

G
Gfellner, B. M. 22
Gianotti, P. 9, 14, 22, 39, 41, 46, 111, 143, 159, 162, 188
Ginot, E. 205
Gold, C. 205
Goldberg, A. 33, 157
Goldfried, M. 7
Goldman, R. N. 82
Greenberg, L. S. 82, 83
Greenson, R. R. 189
grief avoidance 40
grieving process 33
Grossmark, R. 76, 175, 189, 192
ground, concept of 8
Guntrip, H. 32

H
Hartmann, H. 22, 32
Hayes, S. C. 22
healthy narcissism 32
Healthy Self-Actualizing Model 10, 15, 23, 32–35, 36*f*; as companion to Four Quadrant Model 23; compared to Four Quadrant Model 25*f*, 35, 36*f*; definition of quadrants in 27; external actions are challenges to ongoing growth 33–34; grieving of ideal leads to more realistic picture 33; as realistic picture of self-sustainability 34, 34*f*; as safety net 24; spiritual component added to 35; structural design of 24–26, 34–35, 34*f*; symptoms replaced with lifestyle

balance in 26–27; uses in assessment and treatment 37–38
Helms, J. 60
Hill, D. 13
Horner, K. 9, 10, 40, 41, 43, 46
Howell, E. F. 154, 156, 198
humanistic orientation (in psychotherapy) 7

I
implicit bias 61
implicit information processing 12, 13
infant research 6
The Institute for Advanced Psychotherapy, Loyola University, Chicago 4
intergroup relations 61
internal maps 83
intersubjectivity, concept of 13, 58

J
Johnson, S. M. 82
Johnson, S. 75
Joseph, L. 82

K
Kagle, A. 22
Kashdan, T. B. 22
Kernberg, O. 82, 156
Kestenberg, J. 155
Klein, M. 32
Kohut, H. 33, 51
Kuchuck, S. 160

L
LaBarre, F. 6
Lachmann, F. 6, 13, 58
language: complexity of therapeutic exchange 110–111; in creation of meaning 109; entry point to learn about patients' 111–112, 113–114; entry point tracking 119–127; as expression for representation of meaning 108–109; Four Quadrant Model to establish entry points 114–117; inconsistencies in conversation thread 112–113; listening for 111–112; as major tool in talk therapy 109; shift in psychodynamic approaches as communication tool 155; use of in transference 192–193
Lanius, U. F. 204
learned loyalty contracts 50; conceptualization of 50; counter-

transferential experiences and 55–57; couples' communication difficulties and unhealthy 65–71; deeply embedded 53; dismantling 71–77, 146–151; domination at heart of unfair 59; double-bind messages 61–65; healthy 50; marginalization as collective social construction in 59–60; parent's projection of unfinished business onto child 61–65; poorly known or accepted as normal 52; privilege as collective social construction in 59–60; as quid pro quo arrangements 53–54, 55*f*; recognized by observing compulsively driven patterns 51–52; as representation of conflict/tension between wishes and longing 52; in transferential and counter-transferential communications 214–219, 220; unfair 54–55; unhealthy 50, 51; value of working with 51
Leary, K. 192
Levay, A. N. 22
Levine, P. 185
Lichtenberg, J. 131
Listening with Purpose: Entry Points into Shame and Narcissistic Vulnerability (Danielian & Gianotti) 9, 14, 22
Lister, P. 82
Lombardi, R. 178, 179
Long, C. 192
Losada, M. F. 22
losing one's way 2
loyalty 49
the loyalty contract 13–14; *see also* learned loyalty contracts
Lyons-Ruth, K. 6, 13, 58, 89, 157, 204

M
MacKinnon, R. A. 82
Mahler, M. S. 32
Maroda, K. 190
marginalized groups 60–61
Markstrom, C. 22
Marshall, S. 22
McGhee, H. 60
McWilliams, N. 82
mechanistic to holistic shift on human being construct 81–82
mental health treatment 1–2
mentalization 176–177, 185; metaphor as form of 209
Merson, M. 60
Metz, J. R. 22

Michels, R. 82
Millon, T. 82
minority groups 60
Mitchell, S. A. 7, 147
Mitchell, S. J. 32
moment-to-moment tracking 16–17, 129; as form of reflection 132–137; at heart of therapeutic inquiry 151–152; mirroring responses in 142–146, 152; technique of 129–132; as tool in couples therapy 138–142, 140*f*, 141*f*
Morgan, P. 49
multiple theoretical orientations model 3
multiplicity of mind 159
mutuality 58, 198
Myers, V. 192

N
National Institute for the Psychotherapies (NIP) 6
neurobiological development 10; as relational 10
neurobiology 1
neuroscience 8; explicit and implicit aspects of information processes 12–13; as unifying principle in psychodynamic practice 8
neurotic assessment category 82

O
object relations theorists 32
Oedipal complex 7
Ogawa, J. 6
Orange, D. M. 83
Ornstein 33
Othmer, E. 82
Othmer, S. C. 82

P
Pally, R. 6
parent-child relationship 57–58; doer and done to pattern 58; leading to healthy or unhealthy sense of self 57; mutuality in 58; power and surrender conflict traced back to 57–58
Park, N. 22
part-whole analysis 17
patterning 12–13
perfectionism 26
Perry, S. 82
personality splits 39
Peterson, C. 22
practice techniques 3
predilections 7

process dynamics 5–6, 80, 82
psyche: component parts 3; contemporary psychodynamic models to understand workings of 4–5; models of 3–4; organized into integrated or disconnected self-states 160–161; psychodynamic training to consider complexity of 4; splitting off parts of 17
psychic development: healthy upbringing and 21–22; unhealthy upbringing and 21–22
psychic fragmentation 9
psychic organization: defensively driven model 15; evolving lifespan model 15
psychic resilience 22
The Psychoanalytic Situation: An Examination of Its Development and Essential Nature (Stone) 7
psychodynamic case formulation 81–83; affective schemas in 83; categorical assessment in 82; created as teaching tool 82; cultural marginalization in 89–90; emotional process style of patients in 82–83; expansion of scope of 82; formation elements in 82; Four Quadrant Model in 89–92; macro-formulation of a case 83–86; macro-view of a case 84, 86, 86*f*, 87; process mechanics included in 82–83; recast of classical models 90–91; in trauma treatments 87–89
Psychodynamic Diagnostic Manual 22
psychodynamic theory 1; contemporary models 4–5; evolution of 4; integration with clinical observations 3; as major orientation in psychotherapy 7; unifying principles in 7–9
psychoeducation 2
psychological flexibility 22
psychological health measures 22–23
psychological self-continuity 159–160
psychopathology symptoms 39
psychotherapy: cognitive-behavioral orientation in 7; conception of process in present moment 11–12; principles of change 7; psychodynamic orientation in 7; relational dynamic of disruption and repair 8–9
Putnam, F. 158
Putting the theory of the third into clinical practice (Benjamin) 198, 199

R
Rank, O. 7
Rapaport, D. 32
reflexively repeating patterns 39–40; Four Quadrant Model identifies 40
regulation theory 88, 160
Reis, B. 179
relational enactment 191
relationally-based theoretical models 160
relational styles 9–10
resignation: the appeal of freedom 42–43, 45; exquisite sensitivity to being controlled as aspect of 42
resilience 9
Rice, L. N. 83
Riviere, J. 32
Rottenberg, J. 22
Ryan, R. M. 46

S
Schore, A. N. 10, 12, 13, 88, 154, 155, 160, 205
Schore, J. R. 88
self: capacity to distinguish between other and 176; character formation organizing schemas 38; dimensions of to assess health 21; emotional dimension of 144; evolving model over lifespan 15; psychic development of 10; qualities in healthy 39; sacrifice of authentic self to survive 28
self-differentiation 146–147
self-efficacy 22
self-esteem 17; pathological over-compensation and 23
self-idealizing self 39
Seligman, M. E. P. 22
shame, internalization of 8, 23, 89, 90
Sheehy, M. 22
Siegel, D. 209
Society for the Exploration of Psychotherapy Integration (SEPI) 6
solution-focused treatments 2
splitting 156–157; addressing 166–175; catching split-off material incorporating into whole 164–166; as form of dissociative process 156; manifestation of 163–164; motivation for 156–157; as natural developmental state 158; as posttraumatic response 156; transference and 198–199; types 163–164

Stepansky, P. E. 33
Stern, D. B. 51, 109, 152, 157, 160–161, 176, 177, 181, 185, 192, 209–210, 221
Stern, D. N. 6, 11, 12, 13, 58, 147, 176–177
sticking points in treatment 3
Stolorow, R. D. 38, 39, 83, 88, 147, 188, 189
Stone, L. 7
submission 57
subordination 59
Sullivan, H. S. 142, 176
Summers, R. 81
supportive therapy 82
symbiotic-psychotic assessment category 82

T
talk therapy 109; challenges 151–152
therapeutic integration 6
therapeutic mirroring 17, 51
therapeutic relationship 14, 15; mirroring function of 14, 17; transferential enactments in 14
therapeutic safety 11
the Third (Benjamin) 58–59
transference 8, 17–18, 188, 189, 206; aim 191; contemporary psychodynamic views on 189; importance of working with 190–193; as important cutting edge of therapeutic action 14; interpersonalizes patient's organizing schemas 188; non-judgemental belief in 190, 191–192; portal for connecting prior words to present day enactments 191; as powerful leverage for change by therapists 188–189; socio-cultural standpoint on 192; splitting and 198–199; use of language in 192–193

transferential dynamics 5
transferential enactments 188; doubts about statements that may contain 195–196; emotional sturdiness of therapist required 193; entrenched 208–210; listening for entry points 194–195; metaphor to help with 209–214; persistent dynamics and 208–209; sticking points in 209; trust and mistrust are doorways to 195
trauma effects on consciousness 154
Tronick, E. 6, 13, 58, 59, 205

U
Uddin, L. Q. 142
uncovering therapy 82
Uncovering the Resilient Core: A Workbook on the Treatment of Narcissistic Defenses, Shame, and Emerging Authenticity (Gianotti & Danielian) 9, 22, 111
unformulated experiences 175–177; bringing into conscious awareness 77–185

V
Vallerand, R. J. 22
van der Kolk, B. 204
vicious pain cycle 136*f*

W
Wachtel, P. 7, 59, 90, 128
Wallin, D. J. 204
white privilege 60
Wilkerson, I. 52, 59, 60
Winnicott, D. W. 32, 46, 143, 189
Wolf, E. S. 43

Z
Zetzel, E. R. 189